TANTRIC ADVAITA

energizing nonduality

PETER MARCHAND

Copyright © 2022 Peter Marchand

All rights reserved.

Independently Published by Peter Marchand - Belgium.
www.leela-yoga.org

I truly do not believe in something called copyright when it comes to spirituality. Please feel free to share the teachings.
Referring is always nice and useful.

This book is part of a communication project on Tantric Advaita, which has been backed by numerous supporters through the crowdfunding platform Kickstarter.

Cover image by Peter Marchand – the three colored powder drawings in the ash of the ritual fireplace represent the three principal modes of energy, see Chapter 7.

Aum

Gajananam bhootganadhisevitam

Kapitthya jamboo phalasaara bhakshanam

Umasutam shokvinashkarakam

Namami vighneshwar padpankajam

Aum

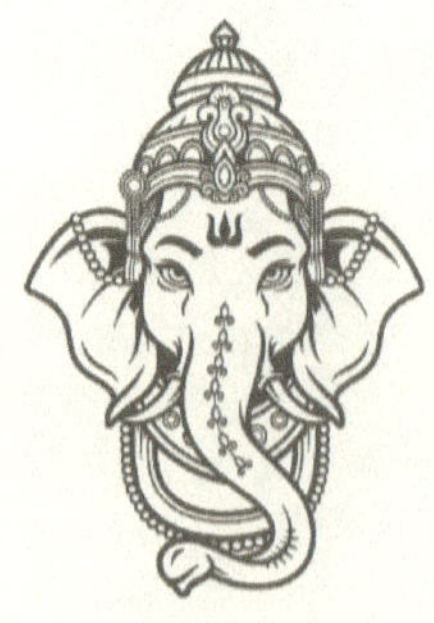

INTRODUCTION

Nonduality means 'not-two', an understanding which is beyond opposites, when everything is perceived as one. Through nondual awareness we can fulfill our desire for peace, which requires us to withdraw our attention from the ever-changing, restless dualities of life. Instead, we focus on an unchanging, nondual, peaceful state of pure being. While this pure being or impersonal awareness has received many names, here we will mostly refer to it as the Self. Nonduality is originally known as *Advaita*, which is the central philosophy of all yoga and meditation. We will fully explore it in the first chapter of this book.

The word *Tantra* is associated these days by most Western people with a more spiritual sexuality[1], while the word basically means to change our energy[2]. *Tantric Advaita* is the knowledge on the nondual energy of the Self, a major but often overlooked aspect of nonduality. *Tantric Advaita* is also known as the central philosophy of the ancient tradition of *Tantra Yoga*[3].

When we think, read or hear someone talking about the Self, we rather easily get a taste of that pure beingness. That taste is experienced as a blissful feeling, which is an energy. But when that great lecture is ended or the book is finished, the blissful feeling easily

---

[1] Tantric sex is a rather small branch of Tantra, where sexual energy serves a spiritual purpose.

[2] Tantra from the root '*Tanu Vistare*' means to 'expand' by 'weaving' together different energies and the knowledge about them. See also Addendum 1 on more related terminology.

[3] *Tantra Yoga* seeks the union of nondual energy and consciousness.

gets lost. And when that particular feeling of pure being is lost, pure being itself is perceived to be lost. *Tantric Advaita* teaches us how to understand and use these changes in order to bring the unique energy of the Self back and keep it.

We can actually never lose the Self, as it is ever in our presence[4], yet we can definitely feel to have lost it. Thus, when the feeling of bliss gets lost, we can try to bring it back by detaching from any unpleasant emotion and focus on our nondual Self-awareness. But if somehow or other we can't do it, then *Tantric Advaita* offers the answers on how to find our way back to the Self by consciously changing our energy. Moreover, *Tantric Advaita* offers many means by which to enduringly maintain the feeling of the Self within our energy. *Tantric Advaita* thus energizes the practice of nonduality, so that we can truly enjoy life in pure beingness.

For most people that try to practice nonduality, when that feeling of pure beingness seems lost, it is not because they don't 'get it'. Intellectually speaking, the Self can be easily understood, even by children. When we lose the bliss, it is also not for lack of trying to hold on to it, because oh boy do we try. The main reason why we so easily lose the feeling of pure beingness is because our energy and thus our feelings are naturally ever changing. Our energy even often becomes blocked in the process and when we feel stuck in an unpleasant emotion, the bliss seems very far away indeed.

The way nonduality is predominantly taught these days, focuses entirely on the non-practice of maintaining nondual awareness. Teachers tend to block the seeker from using any of the other practices[5], which have nevertheless always been part of the ancient

---

[4] More about that in Chapter 1.

[5] This pertains mostly to Western teachers, yet can also be seen to affect practitioners in India, even though the general spiritual community there knows very well the value of the ancient practices because of their continued experiences with it.

yogic traditions. Any alternative route to the Self is generally presented as an illusionary game of the ego, a distraction from the most essential objective.

Modern teachers of nonduality have been mostly influenced by some great *Jnana* teachers[6] of the previous century, with Sri Ramana Maharishi and Nisargadatta Maharaj as the best-known examples. Their emphasis on the direct path of non-doing however addressed a particular imbalance within the Indian culture. People were all too often so much distracted by the more energetic practices, that the most essential practice of maintaining Self-awareness got rather lost[7]. Western nonduality teachers place the same emphasis on non-doing, maybe even with more enthusiasm, in a culture that hardly knows any kind of practice. This logically leads to the opposite imbalance that we are witnessing today. It leaves many practitioners of nonduality stuck into getting it without feeling it. Still some teachers seem to believe that the entire yogic tradition emerged by mistake.

Please understand, I have been inspired by Nisargadatta Maharaj and Ramana Maharishi for decades and I truly admire how modern nonduality teachers have promoted awareness of the Self since many years. It signifies the most important paradigm shift that Western culture has been going through since ages. If I do raise questions in this book about some of the ways in which the Self and the paths have been presented, it is mostly to expand on the subject, letting it further evolve and mature. On the one hand, there are still so many who have no idea about the Self at all and whose attention needs to be withdrawn quite forcefully from the illusion of individuality and duality. On the other hand, there are those who have principally

---

[6] *Jnana Yoga* is the yoga of true knowledge, see also Chapter 10.

[7] Also the Buddha and later Shankara pointed out similar imbalances, so it really is quite an old and naturally recurring discussion. Zen Buddhism also influenced many western nonduality teachers, with a simple teaching that seems opposed to the Tantric ways of Tibetan Buddhism.

understood the sacred gospel of the Self and now need workable ways to live nonduality as individuals. For those, *Tantric Advaita* applied as *Tantric Jnana*[8] is providing many practical methods.

My search for the most essential *Tantric Advaita* teachings was originally triggered by some hints found with Ramana and Nisargadatta. Just like their ancient predecessor Shankara, they understood *Tantric Advaita* quite well and promoted it to some degree[9]. In the words of Ramana himself, if awareness of the Self seems hard to find, one may first try some breathing, some *mantra*, or some other more energetic practice. And if even that does not work to sufficiently calm down, he suggests we might need a holiday. Thus, it became clear that working with consciousness and working with energy, even in the most basic of ways, are complementary. One practice need not exclude the other. They can be alternated or used simultaneously. Awareness of the difference allows for proper balance between these two principal ways of working with the Self. While we focus our awareness on itself, we also harmonize our energy.

Truth be told, in the wisdom gained from my first and foremost teacher Harish Johari[10], there has never been any opposition between working with energy or consciousness. The question only arose years after he left his body. Realizing the complementarity of both approaches made me embark on a mission to

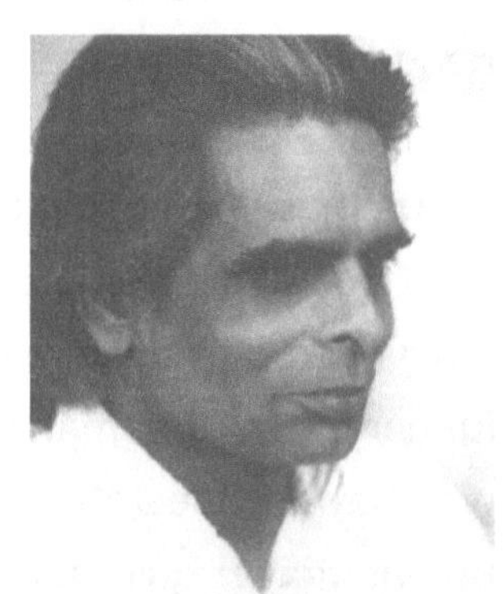

ill. 1. - Harish Johari

---

[8] *Tantric Jnana* is the actual practice of nonduality in consciousness and energy.

[9] See Addendum 3.

[10] I was fortunate to meet Harish Johari, a fabulous author, teacher and artist, when I was only 20 years old. Until he left his body in 1999, I did not listen to any other teacher but him. More about Dada on www.sanatansociety.org.

understand nonduality through *Tantric Advaita* with the utmost possible clarity.

As working with our energy is only truly understood by doing, I became a practitioner of tantric healing about a decade ago. This spiritual and energetic healing practice originates with the Nepalese shamanic tradition[11], which rests upon a foundation of *Tantra Yoga* practiced by the healer. These healings have been remarkably helpful for my students in fundamentally resolving long-standing emotional issues, along with their physical consequences. Whatever I found to be true in this practice, entirely confirmed the teachings of Harish Johari[12]. Nevertheless, it has taken many years before I dared to put the more intuitive awareness of the tantric mysteries that I thus acquired[13], into the rather rational words shared here.

Tantric scriptures are usually relatively secretive, preferring symbolism over reason to communicate the mysteries of nondual energy[14]. What follows is an attempt to bring the original tantric science of nonduality in line with the typical rationality found in modern teachings on nonduality. The most essential understanding in *Tantric Advaita* concerns the seeds or potentials that are hidden within the Self, from which the entire universe manifests. These seeds also offer us the principal energetic methods with which to regenerate the feeling of nonduality and retrace our way back to the Self, which is the central subject of this book. This includes the tantric understanding on how these seeds create the multiple dimensions within the universe, to which our individual souls remain ever

---

[11] As Nepal was never durably conquered by the British, Tantra remained part of mainstream culture, while in India it was more pushed to the fringes of society under British rule.

[12] Even though all of Harish Johari's books touch upon the subject of Tantra somehow, the main reference work is 'Tools for Tantra', Harish Johari, Destiny Books 1988.

[13] See also Addendum 4.

[14] See also Addendum 2.

attached. Thus, the entirety of the yogic tradition is revealed as originating from the Self, bridging the illusion of a gap between nonduality and other practices.

The desire to write about *Tantric Advaita* largely originates from personal interaction with students and also the patients in my spiritual healing practice. In the past years I have experienced a strong increase of people who are principally depressed because they misunderstood nondual philosophy and became stuck in their non-practice. Both teachers and students are responsible for this imbalance. Who doesn't love the doctor who cures all with only one non-pill? Yet the practitioners of yoga postures, breath, *mantra,* or meditation should not be confused about whether all of that is helpful on the spiritual path, or just some distraction produced by the ego. Such confusion is counter-productive, even if people are of course easily distracted.

I hope that with this introduction to *Tantric Advaita*, I can somewhat speed up the passing of this rather natural phase in learning how to deal with our nonduality. Then the beauty of Self-awareness can be truly supported by the entirety of vedic, yogic and tantric science, which is exactly why it was created.

Peter Marchand

NOTE ON THE USE OF SANSKRIT TERMS:

To facilitate the reading for people that are less familiar with Sanskrit, most of the Sanskrit terms have been translated to English, whenever a rather straightforward translation could be found. In those cases however, the original Sanskrit term is also given as a footnote for further reference, as well as for the readers who already know them.

For some Sanskrit words, there is simply no clear translation in English available, because the concept itself does not exist neither in the language nor in the culture. Aside of already quite familiar words such as 'Yoga' or 'Karma', only a few Sanskrit words such as 'Gunas' or 'Kundalini' that seem hard to translate, are thus used within the body of this book.

As the Latin alphabet only has 26 characters, while Sanskrit has 46 of them, the correct writing of Sanskrit words in the Latin alphabet is a subject of much discussion. For example, 'Yoga' is written 'Yog' in Sanskrit, yet the 'g' used at the end of the word includes an 'a' which actually sounds like the 'u' in 'trust'. It's complicated. I have mostly tried to use the characters that seem likely to lead an English reader towards the correct pronunciation.

CONTENTS

p.

1. Nondual Truth... 1.
    • Cosmic Beingness.. 3.
2. Nondual Energy.. 7.
    • Identification.. 9.
    • The Sheaths of Consciousness........................ 10.
    • Changing Our Energy...................................... 14.
3. The Seeds Within the Self..................................... 16.
    • Manifestation.. 17.
    • Seed-Based Practices...................................... 20.
4. The Manifested Seeds... 22.
    • The Sound of Creation..................................... 23.
    • The Mother Matter of Space............................. 24.
    • The Lifeforce of Change.................................. 25.
    • Generating Nondual Energy.............................. 26.
5. Sound... 31.
    • The Sound of Silence....................................... 31.
    • Seed Sounds.. 33.
    • Mantras.. 35.
    • Speech... 38.
6. Space.. 40.
    • The Outer Senses... 41.
    • The Inner Senses... 44.
    • The Elements.. 46.
    • Love.. 54.
7. Time... 57.
    • The Pranic Body... 58.
    • Nine Emotional Energies.................................. 60.
    • The Movement of Prana.................................... 63.
    • The Vibration of Prana..................................... 66.
    • The Storage of Prana....................................... 72.
    • The Polarity of Prana....................................... 74.

- Prana & Desire .... 79.
- The Prana of Consciousness .... 81.

8. Our Soul .... 84.
- The Subconscious .... 86.
- Natural Growth .... 89.
- The Dark Night of the Soul .... 95.
- Feeding the Light .... 97.
- Birth & Rebirth .... 99.

9. Spiritual Dimensions .... 102.
- Vedic Cosmology .... 104.
- Spiritual Travels & Experiences .... 106.
- The Path of Ritual .... 110.

10. Integral Yoga .... 115.
- Paths for the Ego .... 116.
- The Eight Limbs .... 118.
- Tantric Magic .... 120.
- Pitfalls of the Paths .... 122.

11. Keep It Simple .... 126.

12. Good Habits .... 128.
- Daily Rhythm .... 129.
- The Moon Cycle .... 134.
- Other Natural Cycles .... 138.
- Avoidable Habits .... 139.

13. Meditation .... 140.
- Why Meditate? .... 141.
- Learning How to Meditate .... 142.
- Meditation Intention .... 144.
- Relaxation .... 146.
- Concentration .... 149.
- Meditation .... 154.
- Deep Meditation .... 155.

14. Life .... 157.

ADDENDUM .... 161.

ACKNOWLEDGMENTS

Gratitude to the Self, as without it this world would make no sense.

*Gratitude then also to the teachers of Self-awareness,
who have guided me so compassionately.*

*Total credit here is due to the Self, as it is to my very first teacher Harish
Johari, who shaped my understanding as no other.*

*Gratitude to life, allowing this child the time spent in auspicious writing.
Gratitude to the mother and father of life.
Gratitude to those who nurture the love for all three of them.
Gratitude to the yogic and tantric traditions.*

*Gratitude for the special, heartfelt support by
Michael Warshaw, Rebecca Daldini and Régine Deruyver.*

*Gratitude to the many backers from around the world that supported the
'Tantric Advaita' project through the crowdfunding platform Kickstarter.*

*Gratitude to these wonderful people, who provided me with inspiring
feedback on the content of some early versions :
Elena Viklokova, Eric Bennewitz, Evgeny Dziatko, Michael Warshaw, Palatine
Gentils, Pieter Weltevrede, Rebecca Daldini, Rudy Kuhn, Schehrzade Syed,
Shiv Sagar, Stephanie Rees Squibb, Sven Horn and Tanya Gordon Golad.*

*Gratitude especially for the many hours spent
in correcting the English language, aside of giving content feedback :
Chander Mohini, Jan von Meppen, Jason Van Doorn, Natacha Martins,
Régine Deruyver, Rich Dow and Sigurd Andersen.*

Any remaining errors are my own.

1

NONDUAL TRUTH

Dualities are naturally found everywhere in the universe. They appear when a contrast is found between two opposites. In nature we experience summer and winter, night and day, big and small, silence and sound, etc. Many such dualities are also found in ourselves, like in thoughts and feelings, being happy or unhappy, active or inactive, male or female, peaceful or restless. All actions that we undertake in life are somehow meant to change the balance between some of these dualities. We want more of this or less of that, spend endless time thinking on how to achieve it and feel happy or unhappy depending on the results of our actions. We thus naturally live our lives in a state of consciousness that is focused on duality.

Whenever we seek peace however, it can only be found in non-dual awareness, where the restless play of opposites disappears. The nondual Self is our purest conscious beingness, which we can most clearly experience when we stop our thinking process in meditation. Even in that absence of thoughts, we still exist and know that we exist, revealing that consciousness exists beyond thinking. And while thinking always creates dualities, that pure existence seems beyond duality, a true oneness. While our thoughts are ever changing, the conscious witnessing that lies beyond it is experienced as never changing. As it holds no dualities, it cannot change.

The search for the absolute truth about ourselves, the universe and everything, has been narrowed down by yogic philosophy to the search for that which never changes. Whatever changes cannot be absolutely true, as it appears only to disappear, like a mirage in the desert. Only that which never changes can be seen as absolutely true, all else then being at most relatively true. As it cannot change, the Self is seen as the absolute truth. It is who we really are, our true essence[15]. *Yoga* means to seek the union of nonduality[16], so that everything becomes united as one.

Any enquiry into the nature of the universe easily reveals that whatever we find there is ever changing. Likewise, when observing ourselves we find that our body, feelings, thoughts, personality, etc. never stay the same. The only truth that never changes is then found in our pure consciousness, which ever observes whatever happens inside and outside of us. This true beingness is experienced as remaining entirely unaffected by any of the changes that are witnessed outside of it. It is often compared to the screen of a movie theater, which remains white independent of whatever tears or kisses appear upon it. Our pure awareness is in fact our most natural state, yet we tend to identify with what happens on the screen, forgetting that we are the screen. As we are observing the things that happen on the screen of consciousness, we cannot be those things.

This feeling of 'I am, and I know that I am' then is revealed as our most essential existence. Words fall short however when enquiring into the very nature of this existential awareness[17]. We can most easily explain it as not being this or that[18], but to say what it actually is, remains quite impossible. Nonduality is truly beyond words, and yet we can still get a sense of it, while reading between the lines.

---

[15] For a more detailed understanding on the subject of the Self, see also 'The Yoga of Truth – The Ancient Path of Silent Knowledge' by Peter Marchand, Destiny Books 2007.

[16] *Yoga* refers to the root word 'yoke', a wooden bar one carries on both shoulders to unite and balance two opposite objects, such as buckets.

[17] See also Addendum 5.

[18] Known as the practice of '*Neti, Neti*'.

COSMIC BEINGNESS

Qualities are directly related to dualities. The quality of something is expressed as being bigger or smaller than another thing, hotter or colder, more or less dark, etc. When we feel the beingness of the Self, especially in deeper meditation, we cannot say that it is old or young, stupid or wise, happy or unhappy, big or small, dark or light, male or female, etc. It is beyond all such qualities or dualities.

Qualities are what gives a particular form to anything. Having no qualities, the Self is essentially formless. It appears as a void, which is however not at all empty, as it is filled with conscious existence. The formless nature of the Self is hard to grasp for our conceptual mind, which always thinks in terms of dualities, forms and qualities. Yet when mind is quiet, we can still sense this pure beingness existing beyond it, while it remains hard to define it.

As the Self is formless without any particular quality, it cannot change. Only qualities are subject to change. The Self thus seems unaffected by time. We may wonder how something can exist without ever changing and yet here it is, appearing exactly the same last year as it does today. This way, the Self is experienced as eternally unchanging, unborn, unending.

As the Self cannot change, there is also nothing to desire, because we always desire to change something. The Self is desireless and we also cannot desire it to change. And since there is no desire, the Self is ever at peace, just aware of what is. Whenever we are simply enjoying ourselves sitting in the morning sun, it is desire that makes us leave that peace for something else. When we are aware of being the Self, we can easily move beyond desire, except maybe in the desire for peace itself.

Further observance of the Self inside of us brings the clear understanding that the Self is essential to everything we do. Whether walking or talking, thinking or feeling, nothing that we can do is possible without this silent witnessing happening beyond it. We cannot even lift our hand without the Self being the observer of that movement. That observation of what is happening is very much needed in doing anything, because without it we cannot know what we are doing, so then how to do anything? For that reason, the Self is named omnipotent. The Self is not doing anything, but nothing can be done without it. Likewise, it is omniscient, because without it nothing can be known, even if the Self never uses words[19].

Since the Self is thus found wherever something is being done or known, it must be present in everyone. Having found the Self inside of us, we then discover it to exist also in every being outside of us. Behind every eye we meet, that same witnessing must be there, for a pig to do what pigs do, and also for a sunflower or a tree to follow the direction of the sun for example. Hence, we can say that the Self is omnipresent. It exists everywhere in the universe.

When comparing our Self to the Self of a pig for instance, how can we find any difference between them? As our Self has no form and is beyond all qualities and dualities, it cannot be seen as bigger, smarter, happier or in any way superior or inferior to that of a pig. Comparing these two formless kinds of conscious beingness is impossible, as there is nothing to compare them by. We might as well try to compare two invisible clouds. The Self appears as entirely impersonal, devoid of all individuality.

Thus, we can see the Self as the Cosmic Beingness which pervades everything, and in which all are one and the same. There is really only one being looking out from behind a zillion eyes. Therefore, the duality between the individual and the whole is revealed as

---

[19] Part of this power of knowing from the Self also comes as the 'Cosmic Intellect' or '*Buddhi*', available through deep meditation and intuition, which may produce words.

perhaps the most relevant illusion of separation[20]. In essence, there is no 'me' as opposed to 'us'. We are one beingness that witnesses all our various inner and outer forms, whether they are thoughts, dreams, and feelings, or physical bodies, jobs, and environments.

Throughout history, the word 'God' has been most often used to name this Cosmic Being, yet in most people's minds that word is more associated with some supreme being outside of us. As the Cosmic Beingness exists both inside and outside of us, I prefer to use the word 'Self'. That Self is experienced as the illusion of the 'individual' Self, yet it is known to be equal to the Cosmic Self. Looking through a microscope, the drop is not essentially different from the ocean. The ocean exists in every drop.

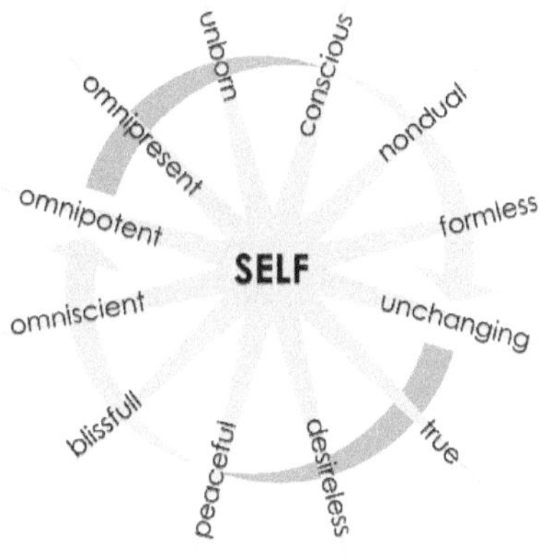

ill. 2. – 'Mindmap' of the Self.

That Self is who we really are[21]. We are all one nondual consciousness, formless and thus unchanging, hence true and desireless, therefore peaceful and blissful, ever omniscient, omnipotent and omnipresent, unborn cosmic beingness. Whatever

---

[20] The cosmic illusion (*Maya*), also known as the divine play (*Leela*).

[21] See also 'The Truth of *Advaita Vedanta*' on youtube.com/youyoga.

individuality we have is not very important compared to the Self and it is anyhow ever changing. We can rejoice in the understanding that we thus ever exist in peace and bliss, yet the question remains how to make this true also in our day to day feeling?

The practice that is most associated with the philosophy of nonduality is to maintain a non-doing, non-trying, non-thinking, nondual awareness. It is the practice of silencing the mind, directly focusing our consciousness on a nondual state of being. This is the path of *Jnana Yoga*[22], where we keep an unrelenting focus on the truth of the Self, a continued dwelling in the silent awareness of the observer. In *Tantric Advaita* we come to the realization that the successful application of this technique can be made easier by simultaneously generating the feeling of nondual energy in ourselves.

---

[22] *Jnana Yoga* is the yoga of true knowledge, see also Chapter 10.

2
NONDUAL FEELING

All we ever really want is happiness. The search for happiness drives all desire and action. We want more of this or less of that, hoping it will make us happier or at least allow us to remain happy. Yet at some point we understand the impermanent nature of whatever happiness we find in the ever-changing phenomena of life. Whatever comes has to go. We can enjoy our ice cream only until it is finished. Whomever we love now must one day die, might otherwise leave us or become less lovable. Tired of running after a kind of happiness that is always followed by unhappiness, the ultimate objective of all yoga and spirituality emerges: to be happy independent of what happens.

The Self is ever beyond the duality of happiness and unhappiness, because it experiences only the never changing, peaceful happiness that is usually referred to as bliss. Living from the nondual Self means ever living in the bliss of the Self, independent of outer circumstances. That is what we are after in yoga, so it pays to always remember that we are in it for the bliss. The Self is the ultimate objective of yoga, maybe not so much because it is who we truly are, but mostly because it gives us the permanent bliss that we really desire. If the Self would only provide us with some empty neutral feeling, nobody would be very interested. Contrary to what some people seem to believe however, the Self is not without feeling. The incredibly true smile on our face whenever we experience the Self is full proof of the bliss that it brings.

The Self is originally defined in scripture as *Sat-Chit-Ananda*, that Being-Knowing-Bliss[23]. The Self is the true beingness, the ultimate reality and the absolute truth *(Sat)*[24]. The Self is also simultaneously experienced as pure silent consciousness *(Chit)*[25]. And last but not least, the Self is also a kind of energy, a blissful feeling *(Ananda)*[26]. That bliss is not just an attribute, but part of the very existence of the Self[27]. *Tantric Advaita* is the knowledge on the essential nature of that energy of bliss. It is the true nondual feeling, the energy of the Self.

As *Sat* or beingness is rather self-evident as long as nondual consciousness and energy are there, the Self is often seen as being 'composed' of *Chit* and *Ananda*, consciousness[28] and energy[29]. Yet the Self truly exists beyond this essential duality. Consciousness and energy may appear as opposites in manifestation, as in thinking versus feeling. Yet, in the Self they are but two sides of the same coin, entirely inseparable. The consciousness cannot exist without the energy, and the energy cannot be known without the consciousness. They are one beingness *(Sat)*.

Especially in modern teachings on nonduality, the Self is most often reduced to consciousness, awareness, the witness, the observer, naming only one half of the pure beingness. That only serves the idea that the best way forward is to focus this awareness or consciousness on itself. Thus, it excludes the energy, the *Ananda*, the bliss of pure beingness, because that would point to the option of

---

[23] Sat-*Chit-Ananda* is also translated as Truth-Being-Bliss or Consciousness-Being-Bliss.

[24] '*Sat*' directly relates to '*Satya*', which means truth.

[25] *Chit* is often written as *Cit*, which is more correct but easily leads to wrong pronunciation, when not actually read in Sanskrit. 'C' without 'h' in English is pronounced as a 'K', like in 'Cave'.

[26] *Ananda* originates from the word '*Nandati*', which means 'he rejoices'

[27] Traditionally, *Satchitananda* is often written as one word, as *Sat, Chit* and *Ananda* are one.

[28] '*Purusha*', which more literally means 'person'.

[29] '*Prakriti*', which also means 'primordial nature'.

working with our energy. That practical option is excluded because it is feared to distract from the more direct path of non-doing, non-thinking, non-trying, etc. by focusing on a feeling of happiness that may or may not be illusory[30]. 'Don't do, just be' is the motto, while all energy work by its nature involves a process of doing, some kind of 'impure' involvement with duality. To state that the absolute beingness is consciousness only and exclude the energy, is however a highly dualistic point of view. All is one in the Self, right?

IDENTIFICATION

To feel the bliss of the Self is essentially a matter of identification, which indeed fully depends on where we focus our awareness. As the 'Father of Yoga' Patanjali[31] famously puts it: 'If the observer stops identifying with the changes perceived in mind, the observer will be itself'. If we identify with what happens outside of us, or in our thoughts and feelings, we will experience the duality of happiness followed by unhappiness. If instead of feeling 'I am this' or 'I am that', we identify with the pure beingness of the 'I am', then it offers us the bliss that we are after.

The ego is then revealed as the main obstruction to living in blissful nonduality, as it is defined as the one who identifies with this or that. We just naturally tend to identify with our body, our age, our feelings, our thoughts, our jobs, our personality, etc. Whatever happy or unhappy feeling we find in these identifications will never last. The logical main practice then is revealed for the ego to identify with the Self only. Whatever happens around us, whatever feeling or thought

---

[30] The light spiritual feeling of *Sattva* (see Chapter 7), which even though it comes most close to the bliss of the Self, is indeed still part of the illusion, as it may come and go.

[31] Sri Patanjali is the ancient author of the world-famous *Yoga Sutras* and often named the 'Father of Yoga'.

comes, whatever ability or connection we find in ourselves, it is then all disregarded as unreal, untrue, a mere illusion.

This is the practice that is known as *Jnana Yoga*, the yoga of true knowing[32]. While it starts with a more intellectual process of understanding the truth of the Self, it ends in true awareness of being the Self. When that understanding and feeling of the Self are present, they only need to be maintained, never again to be lost. Yet that is where the practice of *Jnana Yoga* for most people meets its limitations. In just one second first that blissful feeling and then the knowing can be lost. Daily life seems to bring so many opportunities for that to happen.

The practice of *Jnana Yoga* then prescribes to always return to inner silence to again identify with the Self. Of course, if it can be done, that is always the most direct way to dissolve the illusion of individuality. Furthermore, if thoughts persist anyway, *Jnana Yoga* prescribes that we observe them, question them, discover their illusionary nature to bring them to silence and the direct experience of the Self. Most people however have a hard time keeping this up twenty-four hours a day.

THE SHEATHS OF CONSCIOUSNESS

The reason for our limited control over our ever-changing thoughts and feelings is no big mystery. Especially modern man has predominantly perceived humans as thinking beings[33], which gives us a sense of control in thinking what we want to think. Those who never tried might even believe that to stop thinking must be a piece of cake. The truth is that our thoughts are quite erratic, as they are only

---

[32] See also '*Jnana* Technique' on youtube.com/youyoga.

[33] That distinction between men and animals is actually quite old, with the Sanskrit word for 'mind' being '*Manas*', which in the Indo-Germanic languages lead to the word 'man'.

a reflection of the feelings that lie at their origin. Feelings and thoughts always interact. We are predominantly feeling beings and as such quite complex, as our feelings originate from many different layers of our being.

All matter is made of more or less condensed energy as Einstein taught us, so our physical body is made out of energy. Beyond it however, yogic science reveals that we also have various more subtle energy bodies[34], named the sheaths of consciousness[35]. Every one of these 'bodies' affects the way we feel:

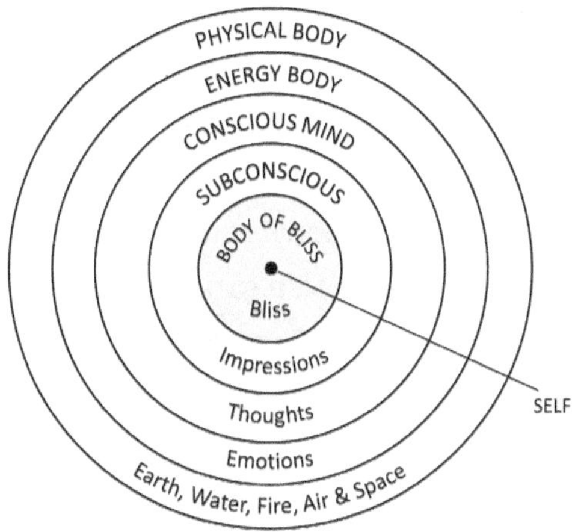

ill. 3. - The Sheaths of Consciousness.

• The physical body[36] mostly influences our feelings and thoughts through the neurotransmitters[37], the nervous system, the brain, and many more energetic systems within the very cells of our

---

[34] See also 'The Koshas' on youtube.com/youyoga.

[35] *'Koshas',* layers as of fine cloth, obscuring the light of the Self.

[36] *'Annamayi Kosha',* the 'food body'.

[37] These 'molecules of emotion' directly affect transmission in the neural patterns of our thoughts and are emotional in nature.

body. If we feel depressed for some time, our body cells will adopt the lethargic feeling. If then we are done with our depression, our body cells may not be. As the physical body is the most dense, it usually slows down any changes in our emotions.

•   The gross energy body[38] is where we actually perceive our gross emotions such as love or anger. Its energy can change in an instant and directly influences the ignorance or wisdom in our thoughts.

•   The thoughts in our conscious mind[39] always have an associated feeling, bigger and smaller likes or dislikes. The two hemispheres of the frontal brain are mostly at play here, producing a rather constant fluctuation between more emotional and more rational thinking[40]. Multiple feedback loops exist between the conscious mind and the other bodies. Fearful thoughts may increase nervousness in the physical body or the gross energy body, yet vice versa such nervousness may also support fearful thoughts.

•   Our most persistent feelings and thoughts originate with the past impressions stored within the catacombs of the subconscious[41], beyond our conscious grasp. Whether it is the animal nature of our reptile brain, the childlike emotional nature of the mid-brain or some deep past life blockages within our very soul, the power with which the subconscious can shake our blissful Self-awareness is truly humbling to the conscious mind.

•   At our very center we find the body of bliss of the Self[42], ever inspiring us towards happiness. It is oftentimes feeling quite out of

---

[38] 'Pranamayi Kosha', the 'body of vital energy', see also Chapter 7.

[39] '*Manomayi Kosha*', the 'body of mind'.

[40] Solar and Lunar thinking, see Chapter 7.

[41] '*Vijnanamayi Kosha*', the 'body of knowledge', also including the cosmic intellect or 'Buddhi' and the principal attachments of the ego or 'Ahamkara'.

[42] '*Anandamayi Kosha*', the 'body of bliss'.

reach whenever too much unhappiness is experienced within the other layers. The actual Self is placed at the 'center' of it, as in illustration 3, even though it exists absolutely beyond any place.

The triggering of thoughts through body, mind and the senses can be rather easily neutralized by turning our attention inside, away from the world. However, the subconscious mind remains the main disturbance of our inner silence. It does not directly produce thoughts, but it rather continuously 'burps' out a kind of wordless feelings[43]. The conscious mind then translates these as concepts that lead to the sentences of actual thoughts through association and reasoning. To stop that process requires quite a lot of mental control. The more we silence the conscious mind, the more the subconscious will tend to fill the emptiness. How to silence the subconscious mind is without a doubt the biggest challenge in keeping the silence and bliss of the Self. For sure, if our subconscious mind is somehow unhappy, it is experienced as a 'pain body' and our bliss will be short-lived. More on working with the subconscious in Chapter 8.

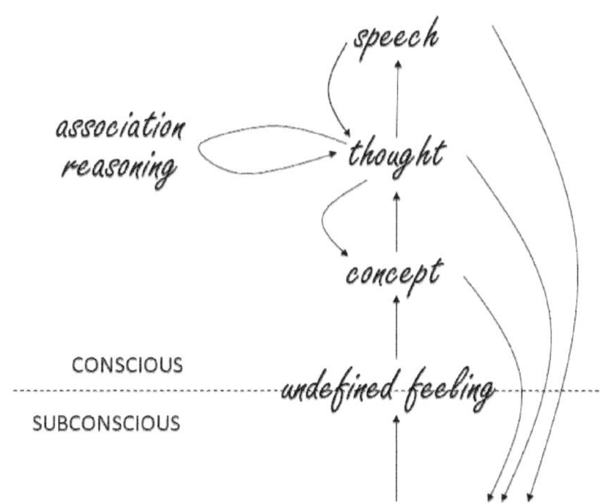

ill. 4. - Interaction between conscious and subconscious.

---

[43] '*Para*', the first of the four modes of speech or '*Vak*'.

CHANGING OUR ENERGY

Whenever our feeling thus loses the bliss of the Self, all we have is the will power of our ego to stop talking to our thoughts, let go of any less blissful emotion, disidentify from whatever attachment caused it, enforce inner silence, and hold on to it whatever happens. Yet our will power itself is a feeling, an energy, ever changing, even if we feel more secure in thinking otherwise. However much we can try to bravely stay 'on top' of our feelings, it may not always be enough if we lack the energy.

Nonduality is therefore not just to be lived within the thinking faculty of mind. If we can't durably feel the bliss, what's the use? What good is positive thinking if our feeling doesn't follow it? What good is not thinking if disturbed again and again by new thoughts originating within our feeling nature? Only if somehow or other we can enduringly generate the energy of nondual feeling, we can really live nonduality. As thoughts and the energy of our feelings are ever connected, energetic control brings mental control. Thus, changing our energy allows us to better control our mind, through which the focus on pure awareness in inner silence becomes so much easier.

It is a matter of common sense. When there is nothing to eat, we can solve the feeling of hunger by disidentifying from the body and turning towards the bliss of the Self. Whenever we are hungry however while food is available, why not eat? Then why not do whatever we can on the different energetic levels of our being, to make it easier to truly feel blissfully beyond any duality in total union? Why not cook real tasty food if the occasion allows it, since we have to eat anyhow? Did not all *Jnana* masters teach us to continue behaving naturally? Are we then also not free to make our own choices?

A more obscure renunciate school in India even chooses to

destroy any harmony in the energy on purpose, as an ultimate exercise in nevertheless remaining with the Self[44]. Yet spiritual progress does not always need to be hard to be real. We have the same natural freedom to change our energy so that nondual beingness becomes a little easier, without of course depending too much on how we feel at any given moment, without too much attachment to our energy. Obviously, this freedom also means that anyone can choose at any time to ignore some feeling and entirely focus on the truth of the Self.

Tantric Advaita energizes the understanding and practice of nonduality by including both the consciousness and the energy of the Self. The pure beingness *(Sat)* is recognized both as an awareness *(Chit)* and as a 'feelingness' *(Ananda)*. The Self is the smiling neutral observer, the blissful thoughtless knowing. It does not just exist, it is conscious, and it has a feeling, an energy.

Tantric Advaita thus defines the beingness of the Self as pure conscious energy. Even beyond manifestation, when there is nothing to observe, this pure conscious energy eternally feels bliss and knows that it does. This feeling/knowing stands unopposed to any non-feeling and non-knowing. It is, without a doubt, it is. And while in manifestation energy always seems to change, the pure, blissful energy of the Self is never changing, just as unmoving and nondual as pure awareness is. They are one. To consciously generate that energy within our feeling may not always be easy, yet fortunately the Self itself holds the very keys to achieve that goal, the seeds of the universe that exist within the Self.

---

[44] The school of '*Agori Sadhus*', famous for drinking alcohol, eating flesh of corpses, etc.

3

THE SEEDS WITHIN THE SELF

In the universe everything is ever changing and hence represents only relative truth, an illusion. It is then obvious that the Self as the only absolute reality must also be the source of this illusion. If not, then this illusion would originate within itself, which would make it an absolute reality[45]. Only the Self is unborn, undying, self-existent, and hence all else is born from the Self. However illusory the universe may be, it must be rooted within the Self[46].

The entire universe is thus nothing more or less than a manifestation of the Self, which then for sure can also be named the Creator. Everything in the universe is but a reflection of it. The Self resides both within and outside of the universe, everything actually being but one. Nonduality must include all duality, otherwise it creates itself a duality between duality and nonduality, between the manifested and the unmanifested, between the universe and the Self. In other words, nondual awareness requires the acceptance and integration of all manifested duality.

Our resistance to accept the universe as part of the truth originates with the search for the Self, where we naturally first tend to look away from the universe to find the Self within. Our Self-realization remains immature however for as long as it disappears when we open our

---

[45] It is truly remarkable how those who are most in favor of regarding the universe as an illusion, often simultaneously ignore its fundamental origin within the absolute reality of the Self.

[46] Likewise, the energy of the universe cannot be born from the consciousness of the Self, if the Self does not in essence contain some energy also, the nondual bliss of *Ananda*.

eyes. If that is still the case, our inner search has not yet been completed. Once we recognize the Self as ourselves both in unmanifested and manifested form, an unconditional love for everything in the world flows effortlessly from our spiritual heart[47].

One moment the wave is a wave, the next it again disappears into the ocean. While it is the most common error not to see the wave as part of the ocean, it is equally untrue to see the ocean as separate from the waves it makes. Thus, in *Tantric Advaita*, the manifested universe is seen as a divine theatre[48], which is manifested from the pure energy of the Self, that has this pure unlimited potentiality. Meanwhile, the Self still exists in unmanifested form. The void is full and ever remains beyond change.

MANIFESTATION

The energy of the Self is truly the most magical of all energies that one can imagine. The seed contains the tree, but the tree cannot be found inside the seed. Likewise, the unmanifested Self contains the potential of all manifested energies in the universe, from ethereal space to the most solid matter. And yet we find no trace of the universe within the Self. *Tantric Advaita* offers us some insight into this mysterious nature of the Self, and how from nothingness things can emerge because they are present within the Self as potentials, often referred to as seeds.

The unmanifested absolute Self somehow holds the potential of the relative, of this manifested universe. The how of it remains a mystery beyond duality and therefore beyond any understanding put into words. Only when we look at how the universe manifests from

---

[47] '*Hridaya*', a *Chakra* in the Heart *Chakra*, also known as the spiritual heart.

[48] '*Leela*', the universal divine play or theatre.

that potential, we can get a glimpse of it. *Sat-Chit-Ananda* or the Being-Knowing-Bliss is the result of that glimpse, representing the main nondual seeds of the manifested universe.

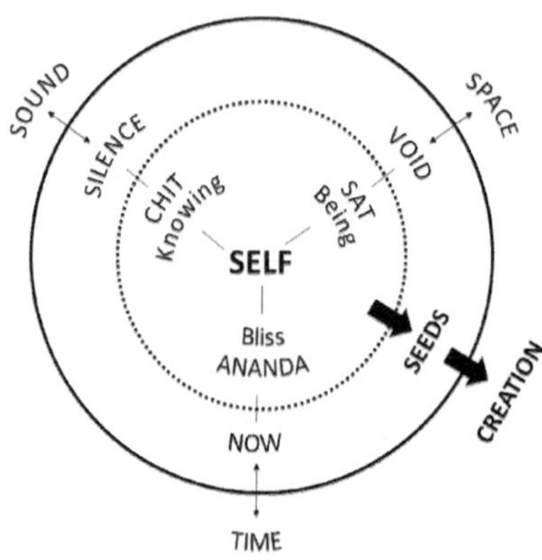

ill. 5. - The Seeds of Creation within the Self.

Chit refers to the pure consciousness which we perceive as a witness, because it observes yet ever remains silent. A witness that speaks and gives an opinion is no longer an impartial observer, not a true witness. The wordless silence is what differentiates the consciousness of the Self from other manifestations of consciousness. Yet when that silent witnessing of the Self is heard as the absence of sound, it is also experienced as a sound, the unstruck sound, the sound of one hand clapping, the sound of an empty cave, the sound of silence. When we hear nothing, we eagerly listen for any sound, because the silence holds or implies the potential of sound. That conscious silence however remains never changing, eternally witnessing without a sound, wordless, without a thought. Hence it is absolutely true as opposed to any sound that appears only to disappear. The sound of the silent *Chit* is the first nondual seed of the universe, holding the potential of all sound vibrations.

Sat refers to existence itself, which can never be questioned because the question itself provides the evidence[49]. It never changes, so it is absolute truth. The absolute Self however exists without form, as a void without any particular quality or property, color or shape. That formlessness is what makes the Self so different from the other things that we experience to exist. We cannot say whether this void is smaller than an atom or bigger than any universe. It is something which is nothing and precisely for that reason, it holds the potential, the very possibility of space and shape. If we were to meet an invisible being, we would naturally wonder what it looks like. When walking in a thick mist that covers everything around us, we still keep looking for some shape or other. The concept of 'zero' cannot even be defined in absence of the potential for some other number. The no-thing holds the potential of some-thing, some shape, some form. Yet the pure beingness without form cannot change, because change is limited to form. Hence the emptiness which is full of beingness is absolutely true as opposed to any shapes or forms that appear in space only to again disappear from it. The full void of *Sat* is the second nondual seed of the universe, holding the potential of space and shape.

Ananda refers to the eternal feeling of this beingness, our true nature which is bliss. This peaceful happiness is self-sustained, unborn, uncreated, uncaused, so it never once began and is never ending. That unchanging nature of the blissful energy of the Self stands opposed to all other energy in the universe, which is ever changing. And because the feeling of the Self cannot change, it is timeless. Only through change we perceive the past as that which was before the change, and the future as that which comes after the change, creating the illusion of time. Time always requires or implies change. *Ananda* is the eternal now, and yet its very timeless changelessness implies the potential of change and hence of time.

---

[49] 'Do I exist' is a nonsensical question, as without the existence of an 'I', the question cannot be asked.

When rain keeps pouring all day, we still wait for it to stop. The clock that stands still, seems poised to start ticking. The absence of change implies the potential for change. Within the Self this potential for change in time is however never changing and thus absolutely true as opposed to any changes themselves which continuously appear only to disappear. The eternity of the now of *Ananda* is the third nondual seed of this universe, holding the potential of time.

The silence of the witness thus holds the seed of sound, the void of beingness holds the seed of space, and the blissful eternal now holds the seed of time (see illustration 5). These are the primary energy potentials from which the universe manifests. To generate the very feeling of the Self inside of us, those are also the primary energies to which we can turn for help.

SEED-BASED PRACTICES

Many teachers of nonduality will promote particular practices that concentrate us on the seeds of the Self, on silence, formlessness and the now. Outer silence can lead to inner silence and the listening to the unstruck sound of silence[50]. We can experience the fullness of presence in our inner space, turning away from the illusion of form created by the senses to the experience of formless existence within[51]. Always staying in the now and disregarding past and future as nonexistent is probably the best-known practice today[52].

In this way, *Sat, Chit* and *Ananda* each offer a direct gateway into the nondual reality of the Self. These are powerful practices based directly upon the nondual seeds of the Self, which come forward in

---

[50] See Chapter 5 and also 'The Sound of Silence' on youtube.com/youyoga.

[51] See Chapter 6.

[52] This is a popular practice thanks to the efforts of Master Eckhart Tolle and his bestselling book 'The Power of Now', see also Chapter 7.

my teachings very often[53]. But they may not be powerful enough when our energy somehow or other has more dramatically moved away from the bliss of the Self.

Our ego is a real drama queen, what to say? That same ego can come to accept that sometimes we are unable to overcome our unhappiness using these quite advanced if somewhat abstract seed-based practices. It is then often experienced as impossible to keep the thoughts silent, to disregard the sometimes painful coming and going of forms to which we feel attached, and to not dwell on our past nor even try to imagine a better future. It is only natural, as people do have lives. Fortunately, the primary energies of sound, space and time that manifest out of these seeds of the Self, are also there to guide us back to the source. They constitute the very essence of the science of yogic practice.

---

[53] See 'Jnana Technique' on youtube.com/youyoga.

4

THE MANIFESTED SEEDS

Basic understanding of the Self has the great advantage of being quite rational and relatively easy to grasp for people with some capacity in abstract thinking. And if thoughts can be silenced for just a few seconds, everyone can have the direct experience of the Self, even if that provides merely a glimpse of the absolute reality of it. This relative simplicity of the Self explains to some degree the popularity of nonduality in these modern times, where rational thought based on experimentation has a status far above all other means of acquiring knowledge.

In tantric nonduality however, we accept the challenge to reveal the mystery of how exactly all things emerged from this 'no-thing' of the Self. The seers discovered that this process starts with the creation of three primal nondual energies within manifestation: Sound, Space and Time. It is a mystery of mysteries, which usually lies beyond our level of direct experience. We can try to grasp it with our intellect, aware however how the illusion created by mind and the senses may stand in the way. The real seeing of the truth behind these mysteries happens in deep meditation when that illusion is dissolved.

If that state of being is still beyond our ability in meditation, we can only rely on what the ancient seers tell us. Those that created the entirety of yogic thought did not just discover the wonderful Self deep inside of themselves, but also the how of its very manifestation into the universe. Some resistance to that unknown territory is natural, as our addiction to understanding can be seen as a means to control our basic fear of the unknown. Few are able and willing to embrace the joy of wonder in facing such uncertainty.

Whatever we may think about that truly mysterious part of the story, the primary energies that manifested out of the Self can be said to be nondual within manifestation[54]. For sure, yogic practices confirm that they can lead us to their nondual unmanifested seeds, in which they are eternally hidden as potentials.

THE SOUND OF CREATION

From the unstruck sound of *Chit* as the silent witness of the Self, the sound of primal vibration emerges, which is generally referred to as *Aum*. As matter to antimatter, *Aum* is the counterpart and product of the silence of the Self. Some prefer to call it the Big Bang.

Of course, the most original sound vibration is not really *Aum*, as *Aum* is just the simplest sound a human mouth can make while opening and closing without any tension in the lips[55]. Yogic science actually refers to '*Visarga*' as a particular breathing sound[56], which is the precursor of *Aum*. Our mouth only parrots as *Aum* the actual buzz sound of creation from the Self, within the Self and around the Self. However it sounds, that primal vibration which we may call *Aum* can ever be heard behind all sounds, is never changing and thus nondual within manifestation.

As the eternal potential of Silence, *Aum* is ever capable of bringing silence to the chattering mind. In *Aum* there is nothing but Self. The power of the sound of *Aum* to calm our emotions is beyond

---

[54] More details in Addendum 6.

[55] This is one reason also why '*Aum*' should never be written 'Om', because to say 'o' the lips have to make a circular shape, while to say 'au' as in 'pause' only requires the mouth to open without any tension in the lips.

[56] The seed sound of the 7th *Chakra*, a voiceless glottal fricative.

comparison. This primal vibration named *Aum* is the precursor of all other sounds. We will dig more deeply into working with Sound in Chapter 5, including the use of silence, chanting, music, tone, beat, seed sounds, *mantras* and speech.

THE MOTHER MATTER OF SPACE

From the void that exists in *Sat* as the true formless beingness of the Self, Space emerges. We usually interpret the word space as empty space, yet both yogic and modern science see space as the most subtle of all matter. Modern science refers to it as 'dark matter' and/or 'dark energy', something that is so subtle that it cannot be perceived and hence is called dark. To this day, its nature remains highly mysterious.

Yogic science refers to it as *Akash*, the etheric space and the most subtle of all matter. It originates from a kind of super element, which is the seed of Space and therefore of all elements[57]. From the most subtle matter of space, all other matter emerges by becoming increasingly dense. Hence from space, the element of air is created, from air fire, from fire water and from water the earth element. In other words, from 'dark matter/energy' to gasses, from gasses to fire, from fire to liquids and from liquids to solids[58]. Every thing known in the universe belongs to one or more of these five elements. Meanwhile formless space remains ever present as the container of all shapes and forms, itself never changing and thus nondual in manifestation.

The matter of space is the mother matter, the dark silence inside a stone. Not only as pure consciousness we are one, we are all children

---

[57] The '*Mahatattva*', the 'great element', including the essence of the 5 elements, as well as the 3 '*Gunas*', mind, intellect, ego and Self.

[58] This ancient Vedic understanding corresponds remarkably well to the view of modern science on how the Earth was formed.

of this mother matter also in our various energy bodies. This mother space creates unity in diversity, giving every manifested being the appropriate space in which to live, just as nature for example offers suitable environments to every species. Giving space is real love, true union, because it is unconditional.

That flexible union of love is where yoga becomes the art of harmony[59], where every one of the five elements is ever again balanced against all others, acquiring its right proportion or place in space. Thus, harmonizing the energies of matter, the void existence inside our inner space becomes easily accessible. More about working with Space in Chapter 6, including the *Dosha*s in the physical body, the inner and outer senses, powerful images to meditate upon in our inner space, and balancing love in our relationships. In Chapter 9 we will also explore the ways to harmonize our public relations within the spiritual dimensions, which are equally related to the five elements.

THE LIFE FORCE OF CHANGE

From the blissful energy of *Ananda,* which is the timeless feeling of the Self, the life force emerges and creates change and time. Change in time means life, from the life of the galaxies, a mountain or a plant to an animal or human being. Change is the magic of the life force, which we principally experience as the energy that keeps us alive. It is however also discovered as the primary power behind all change in the universe, active within the tiniest of particles. It is the ever-changing, ever pulsating nature of the primary energy of time emerging from the Self and known in yogic science as *Prana.* While

---

[59] '*Dharma*', often named by Harish Johari as the most essential practice and attitude for durable spiritual growth. All '*Adharma*' or that which goes against *Dharma*, leads us away from the Self, because it goes against the law of Love, which is the law of union of the Self.

its nature is ever changing, it is also never changing, ever present as the energy of change, time and life. Thus ever creating change within the universe, the very life force of change remains ever present and is nondual in nature within manifestation.

The sciences related to the life force are highly varied, because of this ever-changing nature. Many ways exist to categorize these fluctuations in order to work with the life force. *Prana* can be seen as a kind of subtle primordial electromagnetic energy, while it also has less subtle manifestations such as the electrical currents that run through our nerves or the heat released in meditation as a result of relaxation. Yet yogic science very much emphasizes the more subtle channels of these energies[60] within our more subtle energy bodies, creating a large number of important energy centers[61].

Related practices are using breath and many other means through which our vital feeling can be most easily brought back to the bliss of the Self. The many tools that relate to the various forms of *Prana* are discussed at length in Chapter 7, including the *Pranic* body, the vibration of *Prana*, the storage of *Prana*, the polarity of *Prana*, the energy channels and centers that affect our desires, and the famous transformational lightning power of *Kundalini*.

GENERATING NONDUAL ENERGY

Manifestation from the Self thus means the movement from the unstruck silence to the Sound of *Aum* and all other sounds, from the presence as void to all matter of Space, and from the timeless bliss to the illusion of Time created by the life force of change. In yogic practice we close the gap with the unmanifested *Sat-Chit-Ananda* by

---

[60] '*Nadis*', see Chapter 7.

[61] '*Chakras*', see Chapter 7.

reversing this process. We can produce the sound of *Aum* to create silence, balance our energy in gross matter and form to generate the lightness of formless space or *Akash*, and change the energy of our *Prana* to the neutral vibration that produces timelessness. It is from these most essential practices that the entire yogic tradition emerged to help in bringing our energy and feeling more closely to the bliss of the Self.

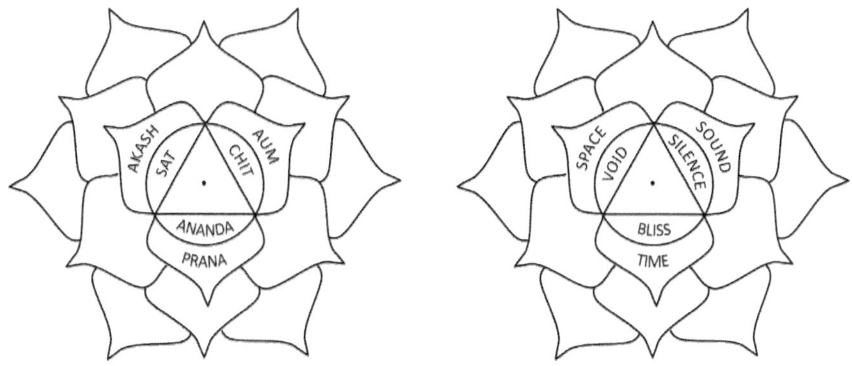

ill. 6. - The Lotus of the Manifesting Self.

Another reason why nonduality is so popular these days is because the most directly related practice is fairly simple to understand and seems to require little effort. It is a non-practice, a non-doing, a presumably simple withdrawal into the observer mode of the Self. However wonderful and relaxing, this practice is in truth far from simple, especially if we want to keep it up for more than a few seconds. Intellectually it is simple to grasp, yet to believe it is easy-peasy in practice equals ordering frustration from the menu, especially if the energy is somewhat disturbed.

As energy always changes, taking on many different forms, the techniques by which nondual energy can be generated are quite diverse and complex. To master them requires effort and some real concentration power, which is relatively poor in modern society. Fortunately, we only need these techniques in as far as we have a concrete need for them. And we definitely do not need to master all of these techniques to be able to generate a lasting nondual feeling in ourselves. Fully mastering only one of them[62] might even suffice, as all nondual energies are naturally intertwined. Transforming one or a few, we can affect all others.

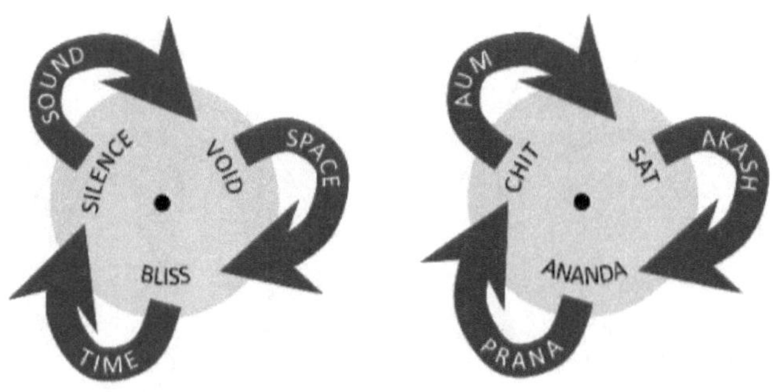

*ill. 7.- Eternal Play between the Seeds of the Self
and their Primary Manifestations.*

Sound, Space and Time are entirely interdependent. To mentally separate them is only needed to understand and utilize them. In *Tantric Advaita*, Time as the life force is said to be the first born when the universe manifests from the unmanifested. This was the first change and hence the creation of Time[63]. Consequently, the universe is born from the *Ananda* or bliss of the Self, which holds the potential of life, change and time. Then Time, *Prana* or life triggered the Sound of *Aum* out of the unstruck sound of the silent consciousness *Chit.* And finally, *Aum* created Space from the void existence of the Self or *Sat,* as the mother of all matter in the universe. All this continues to

---

[62] See Chapter 11.

[63] In Tantra, this divine manifestation is also named 'Kali', who is '*Adiya*', the first-born.

happen as manifestation evolves, space holding life, life creating sound, sound generating more space, an endless spiraling motion around and from the Self (see illustration 7).

Therefore, when in *Tantric Advaita* we seek the pathways to enhance in ourselves the blissful energy of the Self, then the life force that is born from the bliss of Ananda is not the only energy with which to work. Both the sound that emerges from the silence of the witness consciousness, as the mother matter space that originates within the void of pure beingness, equally manifest as particular nondual energies that support the bliss of the Self.

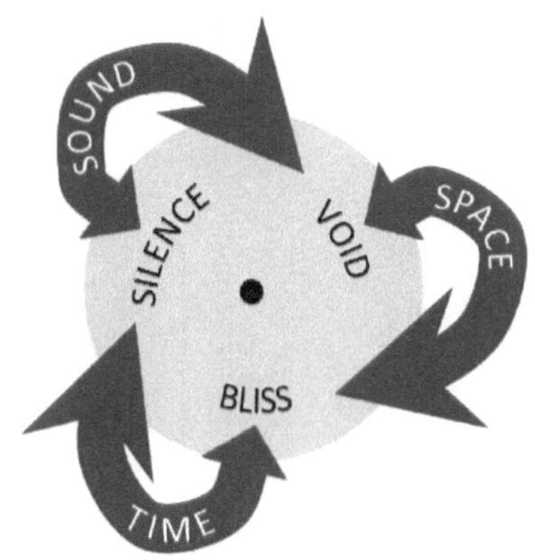

ill. 8.- Interaction between Practices and the Seeds of the Self.

Compared to illustration 7, the above illustration has been slightly altered to show how this interaction works when the words Sound, Space and Time are seen as 'practicing with' Sound, Space and Time. Working with Sound not only leads to silence - it also affects emotional detachment, increasing identification with the void beingness of the Self. Balancing the various manifestations of the Space element not only generates that same detachment – it also brings a rather more physical feeling of contentment and well-being that stimulates connection to the bliss of the Self. Finally, working with the life force of time through breath, etc. not only brings more of that bliss – it also calms and purifies the mind so that the silence of the Self can be heard more clearly. It all works together, in ever more intricate ways, and so any related practice will benefit from a more holistic approach.

The three primary energies of Sound, Space and Time, or *Aum*, *Akash* and *Prana*, are one. In the ancient traditions we can see how their use is often combined to make the practices more powerful, more complete, more transformational. It means that yogic practices and sciences are not so easily arranged along this primary trinity of manifested energies, as many are in fact overlapping and interacting. In the following three chapters, we will nevertheless give it a try to thus categorize them.

5

SOUND

The primary energy of Sound, which emerged from the silent knowing or *Chit* aspect of the Self, is the key to inner silence. The practice of inner and outer silence is the beginning and end of all yogic techniques that use the primary energy of sound. In between, the power of sound vibration to change different energies in ourselves helps us across the pond of our sometimes-turbulent emotions. *Aum* and many other sounds can enduringly lead us to the silence of the Self, which holds the truth of knowing. Moreover, when sound and silence are alternated, the sound emphasizes the silence, making it almost literally audible. To hear the silent space behind all sounds around us, naturally we keep silent inside.

THE SOUND OF SILENCE

Hence many techniques using sound in silence have been developed: the slow and peaceful chanting that includes many pauses, some breathing techniques such as the humming bee breath[64], and the fast rhythmic use of sound produced by voice, drums, bells and other instruments. Many can easily find the inner silence simply by making a sound and then silently listening to the silence that follows it. When thoughts reappear, again some sound can be used to attract the attention to the sense of hearing and its

---

[64] *'Bhramari Pranayama'.*

inherent silence. Also more continued use of sound creates a drone-like effect that generates silence inside, such as in Shamanic drumming.

Sound is very powerful, because the sense of hearing relates to the element of space[65], which is the origin of all elements and ever present within all elements. Therefore, through sound we can affect all elements out of which our body is made. Also in western science the universe is found to consist entirely of vibrations that can be measured as sound frequencies. One might say that the sound vibrations of the energies of our body so much want to be heard, that keeping silent is really difficult. Using sacred sounds to harmonize our sound vibrations can remedy that. Sound has been shown to change even the molecular vibrations in our body, enhancing the capacity of molecules to interact with each other through biochemical processes.

Overtones are produced at a different frequency than the main tone that we are making and are known to have an even more profound effect on our sympathetic nervous system. They may regulate our breath, digestion and many of the other processes that are happening automatically in the body. While the pronunciation of a *mantra* for example mostly influences the left hemisphere of our brain, the tone and melody affect the right hemisphere. When all aspects of our entire being are chanting in harmony, deep inner silence follows.

Chanting *mantras*, spiritual songs and basic sounds such as *Aum* alone or in a group[66], has been found by many to produce long lasting bliss and inner silence. Slow chanting with many silent moments in between is most suitable when chanting alone, thereby relaxing mind

---

[65] See Chapter 6.

[66] Known as '*Kirtan*'.

by reducing the breathing and heart rates. Faster chanting is easier for groups because the beat keeps everyone on track. It may bring a feeling of trance followed by a deep relaxation afterwards through basic exhaustion in concentration[67].

Singing requires a particular kind of breathing, with side effects on our life force that correspond to certain ancient yogic breathing techniques[68]. The Indian musical scene has been much influenced by the yogic sciences of breath and sound, leading for instance to the preference for gliding notes to produce particular levels of emotional stimulation and relaxation. Intuitive singing from a kind of devotional silence is a particularly interesting practice of channeling. It quite directly teaches us how to let the Self inspire our every word and action[69].

SEED SOUNDS

Whatever sound we sing, speak or think will influence our energy. The Sanskrit alphabet is unique in this respect because every sound used has a particular meaning which is associated with the particular effect it has on our energy centers. For example, if we use a sound which creates an energy that makes us feel more courageous, then the meaning of that sound in Sanskrit will also be for example the word 'courage'[70]. When a word is composed of different sounds, the meaning of it will reflect the combined energetic impact of the sounds it is made off. Sanskrit is therefore a language which is literally creative.

---

[67] I often invite people for 2 hrs. of non-stop *Gayatri Mantra* trance chanting.

[68] '*Pranayama*', see Chapter 7.

[69] This is the essential practice of '*Dhrupad*' singing.

[70] To translate basic sounds is not always that simple though, as history made its mark on it.

While *Aum* is the seed of all seed sounds, many other powerful seed sounds have thus been discovered. This magical yogic science of sound was not established in the normal waking state, by using certain sounds and then experiencing their effect on our energy and emotions. Given the many factors that affect our feelings, that would be quite an impossible task. This science was developed through deep meditation by the so-called *Rishis*, the ancient seers of vedic culture, the yogis of ancient times. The word '*Rishis*' comes from the word '*Richa*', which particularly points to essential divine sound energies[71]. In that way *Rishis* are not only 'seers' but also 'listeners'. The essential sounds of the Sanskrit alphabet were heard and energetically experienced by these yogis in deep meditation[72].

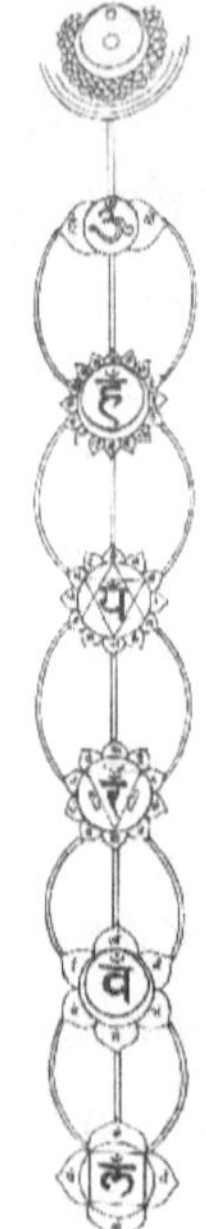

ill. 9.

Chakra sounds

The science of sound for example includes the knowledge that vowels are less related to the gross energy of the body than consonants. They are therefore most potent in affecting our more subtle bodies. Consonants are found to be more effective in changing the energy of the physical body and the gross energy body. The *Rishis* even created the so-called body of sound[73], mapping different sounds within the subtle energy centers of the body. The repeated use of seed sounds[74] to affect different energy centers is a particular yogic science related to *Kundalini Yoga*[75]. This knowledge can be found hidden within the construction of the more

---

[71] Recorded already in the oldest of scriptures, the verses of the *Rig Veda*.

[72] This happens in the state of '*Samprashnad Samadhi*'.

[73] The '*Mantra Purusha*'.

[74] '*Bija Japa*', related to the *Chakras* or also often in the form of '*Nam Japa*', reciting the name of some divine energy, ideally with only one syllable.

[75] See Chapter 7.

tantric *mantras* as well. We literally have thousands of energy centers in our body, which all generate different desires and attachments, leading to often persistent thoughts and feelings. The life force or *Prana* interacts with the elements within the body through these centers, producing certain sound vibrations and the related desires. Even if we only look at the seven main *chakras*, tantric science discovered no less than 57 different seed sounds affecting distinct aspects of these primary *chakras*[76]. Through the use of these seed sounds, our basic desires can be harmonized[77].

MANTRAS

Also the ancient *mantras* are the product of deep meditation, not just poems created in the normal waking state. *Aum* is the mother of all *mantras*, directly producing the energy of the Self. Hence all *mantras* designed to enhance the feeling of the Self start with *Aum* and end in *Aum*[78]. The ancient *mantras* are used as particularly powerful spells which fundamentally change our energy. One splendid example is the famous *Gayatri mantra*, which works on 24 different energy centers through 24 syllables[79]. It has a fantastic effect on how we feel, and easily in that way, brings us so much closer to the Self and deeper meditation.

Mantra Yoga is a standard ingredient of just about any spiritual tradition and a major branch of *Tantra Yoga*. *Mantras* are energetic sound postures for the mind. The energetic effect of repeating certain

---

[76] For audio, listen to 'Sounds of the Chakras', Harish Johari, Destiny Recordings 2004.

[77] See Chapter 7.

[78] Most *mantras* that start with *Aum* are usually not written as ending in *Aum*, because *Aum* comes again with the *mantra* recited next. However, when using such a *mantra* only once, it is best to also use *Aum* at the end.

[79] See also 'Gayatri Mantra Meditation' on youtube.com/youyoga.

sounds in the mind is extremely effective in transforming ourselves. It allows us to work with the subconscious mind, calming for example the reptilian brain with sound like a snake charmer would. Some *mantras* like the *Gayatri Mantra* are specifically designed to enhance Self-awareness, while others may be used for example to reduce anger or fear, generate feelings of love and joy, remove particular attachments, etc.

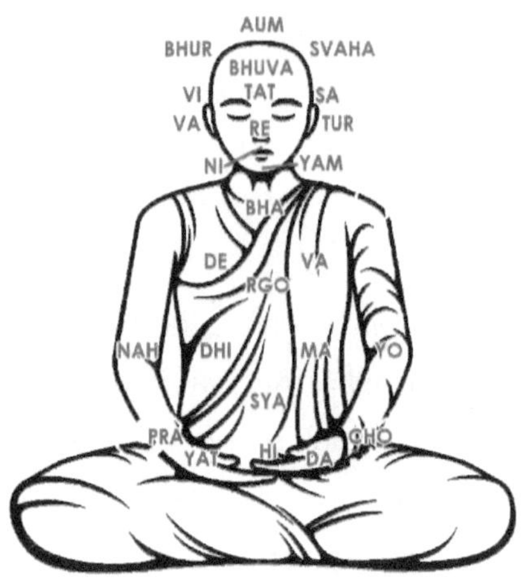

ill. 10. - Energy Centers harmonized by the Gayatri Mantra.

Next to *Aum* which is directly related to the creative power of the Self, other highly potent sounds have been connected to particular aspects of that power, such as *Hreeng, Kleeng, Hum, Bram,* etc. One might say that they produce a particular flavor of the peace that *Aum* represents. *Aum* produces the most gentle and subtle kind of peace, while some of these other sounds for example create a kind of peaceful strength that may be more resistant to whatever emotion may threaten our peace.

In *mantra* meditation, *mantras* and seed sounds are used as objects of meditation. Since sight and hearing are the most active senses in the minds of human beings[80], using one of these in concentration is very effective to engage mind[81]. Compared to the meditation on some more abstract concepts such as 'the I' or 'the now', *mantras* clearly offer more concrete and engaging objects for mind to hold on to, but there is more.

While being used as any other object of meditation, their particular energetic effects on our entire being may support a more meditative state. When chanted out loud, the main effect is in the physical body, the gross energy body and the conscious mind. When recited inside, the same sounds will more directly affect the deeper subconscious mind. This ancient practice has proven to bring long-lasting results, so that when the meditation is finished, life can be lived with much more Self-awareness, detached attachment, peace and bliss. Mantras are also powerful tools to harmonize our public relations in the spiritual world, as we will discuss in Chapter 9.

Aside from the use of *mantras* in meditation, they can also be repeated during daily life[82], whenever our activity does not require much thinking, such as in driving, cleaning, cooking, etc. Whether sung out loud or recited inside, using *mantra* in life will deeply affect our energy. The more we use them, the more their energetic pattern will vibrate within our entire system and gain power. The neural pattern of the *mantra* in our brain will become ever stronger and the related biochemical and energetic patterns will become habitual. Finally, even just reciting a *mantra* only once may have the power to immediately change an unpleasant mood.

Writing *mantras* is another powerful practice, simultaneously concentrating and relaxing, with both the auditive and the visual

---

[80] Dogs for example would probably more easily concentrate on some smell.

[81] To cover both hearing and sight, we can use *mantra* in combination with *yantra*, see Chapter 6.

[82] This practice is known as '*Japa*'.

hemispheres[83] being affected. *Nada Yoga* is another tradition worth exploring, entirely focused on inner sound vibrations.

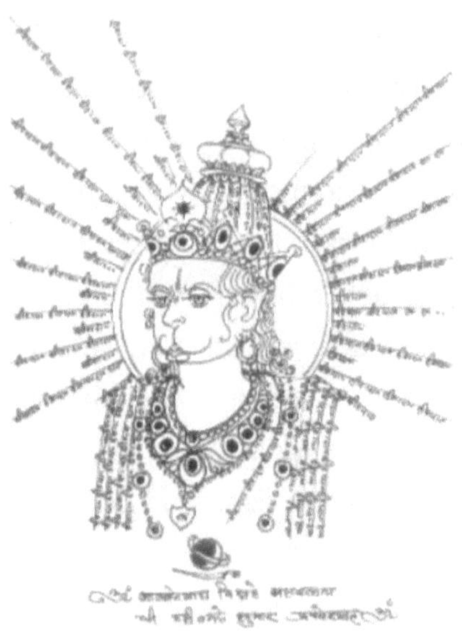

*ill. 11. - My teacher Harish Johari created this
kind of 'written mantra' for Hanuman every day.*

SPEECH

While the energetic effect of *mantras* is much more relevant than their meaning, many of them have profound significance to our comprehension. In the ancient yogic tradition, much emphasis was laid upon memorizing certain *mantras* and other spiritual poetry. This was not only a means of safeguarding the knowledge at a time where no books yet existed. The very repetition used to memorize this

---

[83] See Chapter 7.

knowledge also engraves it upon ourselves as neural, biochemical and energetic patterns, that will continue to affect our thoughts and feelings.

There is power in words and in thinking truth. Even if words are just concepts based on other concepts, better to have relatively organized and positive thoughts, rather than meaningless and negative thoughts. Armed with words of truth, negative thinking can be taken by the tongue. Seeking the 'I am' in every thought, the illusion of any thinking that goes against the law of union can be revealed. Are we talking about 'you' or about 'us'? True words even have the power to stop all thought and lead us to silence. Such words are usually not the product of reasoning. They come as pure intuition, a 'seeing' of truth turned into sound.

Thinking is nothing but internalized speech, and we are then also the sounds that we think. Repeated sound frequencies, including their meaning, thus have great powers of transformation. This wisdom teaches us to be watchful for untrue words that we frequently speak or think, as they are not without consequence. To share our insights into the truth will likewise generate it around us.

6

SPACE

The primary mother matter of Space, that emerged from the void beingness or *Sat* aspect of the Self, offers many opportunities for balancing imbalances that affect our feeling of bliss and detachment. This mostly pertains to the elements within our physical body as well as to the sensory input which we receive from our environment.

Respecting our body as a temple made of five elements is the correct attitude to remove it as an obstacle from the path, however much we can think that we are not the body. The elements are regarded as sacred in *Tantra* and worshipped at the start of many rituals.

Balancing the elements and the related senses brings peace on the most material level of our existence. That much less of a distraction allows us to more easily detach from our forms and connect with the inner space of our truly formless being. The more we are impressed by the illusory reality created by the senses, the more the feeling of separation, aka the ego, persists. The more we identify with our formless essence, the more we can feel connected to all forms and beings in

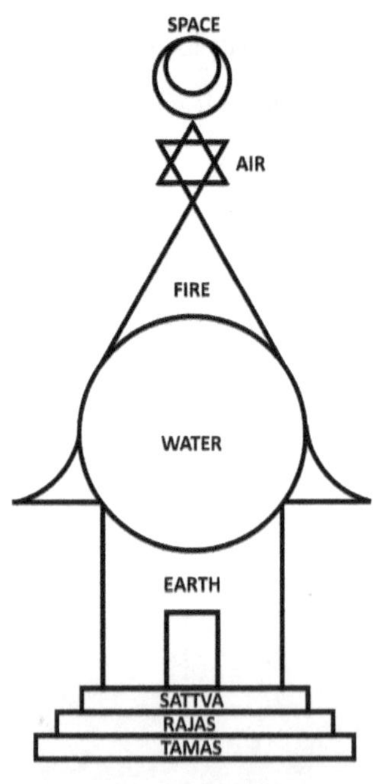

ill. 12. - The Temple (Stupa) of the Body.

the Space of the universe. And the more we feel connected, the more our power of perception is purified, and all sensory input is perceived as blissful[84]. It is the foundation of all true art and of unconditional love also.

As the elements have gradually evolved out of the Space element[85], Earth as the densest element holds all other elements. Water includes all elements except Earth. Fire incorporates Air and Space. Air is contained by Space and Space is just Space. This insight is essential to work with the elements.

	Earth	Water	Fire	Air	Space
Earth	x				
Water	x	x			
Fire	x	x	x		
Air	x	x	x	x	
Space	x	x	x	x	x

Table 1. - Elements contained within the elements.

THE OUTER SENSES

The five elements that emerged from the void of the Self are experienced through the five senses. The senses are actually the very seeds of these elements. We experience the Earth element through all senses including the sense of smell, while all other pure elements have no smell. The Water element comes to us through all senses except smell and including taste, while the remaining elements have no taste, as the tongue needs water to taste anything. The Fire element is experienced through the senses of touch, hearing and also sight, while Air and Space remain invisible. As we can feel the wind on our skin, Air is experienced through the senses of hearing and also

---

[84] The more spiritual interpretation of 'Beauty is in the Eye of the Beholder'.

[85] See Chapter 4.

touch, while Space cannot be touched. Finally, sound is known to also travel through the dark matter of 'empty' Space, which is the only way how that element can be experienced when no other elements are present, as in outer space.

	Earth	Water	Fire	Air	Space
Smell	x				
Taste	x	x			
Sight	x	x	x		
Touch	x	x	x	x	
Hearing	x	x	x	x	x

Table 2. - Experience of the Elements through the Senses.

To find that silent inner space inside, we need not just to close our eyes. We need to stop looking, otherwise some lightshow will always remain visible behind the eyelids. Withdrawal of the senses[86] is a matter of attention, the turtle withdrawing into its shell. We have no way to entirely stop hearing if we are still listening. While the senses of touch, taste and smell are less important to us humans, the same applies to all. Meditating in the dark, putting numbing ash on the skin, plugging the ears with a cotton ball, rinsing the mouth with water, and burning incense when meditating, are easy ancient ways that may be quite helpful.

Consciously withdrawing the *pranic* energy from the senses is another method, but that is mostly a matter of attention, as *pranic* energy follows our focus[87]. When we turn inside, the life force naturally follows. In this way, fully concentrating on an inner object automatically removes the attention from the outer objects.

Too many people have been led to believe that meditation means to objectively observe the sensory input from the environment, as well

---

[86] '*Pratyahara*', literally going against what is incoming.

[87] See Chapter 7.

as any thoughts or feelings. This technique, also known as mindfulness, still leaves the mind full of impressions. Such practice is merely a very good preparation for meditation. In actual meditation, we have no more sense of sitting somewhere and really inhabit our inner space, empty of all outer sensory activity.

The conscious mind is our main interface between inside and outside. There we process all incoming information from the senses through thoughts and feelings, affected also by the responses of the subconscious, based on past experiences. Our true inner space however lies far beyond the conscious and subconscious minds. That is where real deep meditation leads us, to that void beingness of the Self.

When our senses are over excited, withdrawing our attention from them becomes more difficult. When our daily sensory input is calm and pleasant, a strong feeling of security is produced by the senses, an 'all is well' message from these primary watchdogs. Satisfying, harmonizing and relaxing our senses has always been part of the yogic lifestyle. Soothing but low vibrating sounds, pleasant colors in rounded shapes, nice subtle earthly smells, sober yet creatively satisfying foods, natural fabrics on oily skin, etc. can all help to calm our senses and nerves. Likewise, whenever possible we can avoid sharp and high tones, overly bright or dark colors in rectangular shapes, strongly arousing or disgusting smells, junk foods with imbalanced strong tastes as well as uncomfortable fabrics and dry, irritable skin. Without allowing too much dependency, when the occasion arises, we make sure to enjoy and share good food, nice music, natural beauty, a great hug, not forgetting to smell that rose we just passed by.

Modern society has made sensory overload the norm, just to serve the economy. Especially modern media produce ever intensifying sound and light shows to keep the attention of their consumers. To allow for real meditation, some media fasting is essential, especially for people who already experience having become overly sensitive to sensory input. In such cases the senses need to be purified and relaxed prior to any meditative practice.

THE INNER SENSES

The outer sense organs deliver their information to the inner senses of the conscious mind[88], where the actual experience of sensory input is taking place. The inner senses allow us to visualize relaxing sensory objects in our mind, without needing those objects to exist outside of us. To hold the inner space at first is easiest if we can place some form inside of it. Thus, visuals are used as objects of concentration in meditation.

Our more rational left hemisphere is mostly engaged by words, while the more emotional right hemisphere is more thinking in images[89]. Using words and images simultaneously in meditation is a very powerful tantric practice that may be very useful to overcome difficulties in concentration[90]. A wide variety of powerful archetypal symbolic images such as a flame, a lotus, the sun, the *Aum* symbol, etc. can be used. While the actual meaning of such visuals may aid in our motivation to concentrate, tantric science has developed very particular visual objects that have energetic effects similar to those of *mantras*.

Such *Yantras* are geometrical patterns based upon a deep understanding of the effects of various shapes and colors on our energy. Just the practice of having a *yantra* in a dominant place in our

---

[88] The '*Tanmatras*', responsible also for all sensory perceptions in dreams.

[89] See Chapter 7.

[90] Meditation is often disturbed by thoughts that manifest either as words or as visuals. Using sound and image in meditation blocks both these entry points for thoughts.

home will have a similar effect as for example regularly playing some meditative music. They all have a central dot[91], which is the focus of concentration and the essence of the *yantra*. Some people are able to immediately picture in their mind a complete *yantra* with all the circles, squares, petals and colors. They are usually good at drawing too.

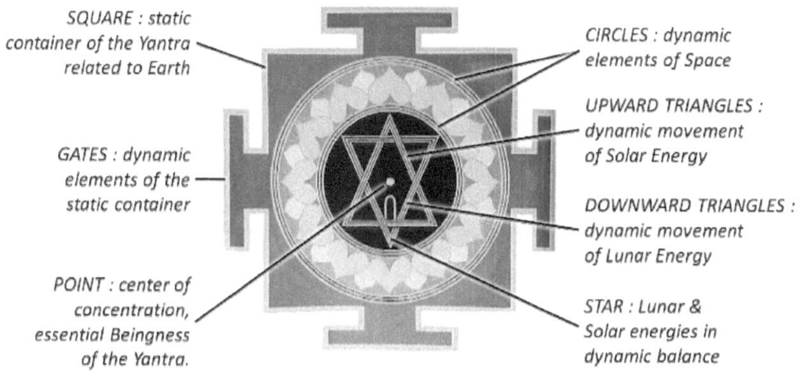

ill. 13. - Examples of the 'Grammar' of Yantras.

For most people, to really get to know the *yantra* they first have to paint it. A *yantra* is painted from the outside to the inside, so the last thing one adds is the central dot. Then also in our mind we reconstruct it that way. The outer shape is usually a square, but with some gates added. This way the square does not become too square and thus less static. The square is needed so that we can focus our attention within a certain field. *Mandalas* for example are circular, which is the most dynamic form. The circle is an expansion of the dot, so to keep a circular image stable in our mind is very hard. It always tends to grow bigger. Inside the square usually one or more circles are drawn, contained by the square. Inside the circles there are often

---

[91] The *'Bindu'.*

triangles, which create an upward or downward movement of the energy. The dot in the middle represents the most essential energy of the *yantra* and ultimately the Self.

The effect of each color used within these geometrical forms is also very important. When we visualize such a color, it produces the complementary color inside of us, and that is the color that we are actually seeking in terms of effect[92]. In the final stages of *yantra* meditation only the dot remains, which then naturally expands into our deep inner Space, inviting us to dive in.

THE ELEMENTS

Yogic science provides many ways to remove the senses from their outer objects and lead us to the formless Space of the Self. However, we are still the ones who need to make that effort, and the experience is that our other desires easily get in the way. These desires are primarily created through identification with imbalances in the five elements of our body, while the desire to meditate can be seen as the desire to move beyond the elements. Balancing the elements in the physical body then becomes a major way in which we can facilitate the withdrawal from the senses, which are ever providing distracting input from the elements.

Identification with the Earth element, which creates the form of the physical body, leads to the basic desire for security in terms of money, possessions, health, etc. Identification with the Water element, in which we experience our gross emotions as sensations through the intermediary of neurotransmitters, hormones, etc. [93] leads to the basic desire to pleasure mind and the senses. Identification with the light of

---

[92] Full details in 'Tools for Tantra', Harish Johari, Destiny Books 1988.

[93] The blood plasma, the cell plasma and also the cerebrospinal fluid.

the Fire element, in which we feel exposed to the view of others, leads to the basic desire for social status. Identification with the Air element, which connects us to others as the prime carrier of the life force, leads to the basic desire for unconditional love and togetherness. Identification with the Space element, which allows us to observe things from a distance, leads to the basic desire for understanding. Identification with the source of all elements leads to the basic desire for enlightenment in detachment from the elements.

ELEMENT	PROPERTY	DESIRE
Earth	Form	Security
Water	Sensation	Pleasure
Fire	Illumination	Status
Air	Connection	Love
Space	Distance	Understanding

Table 3. - Desires of the Elements related to their Basic Properties.

If our meditation is disturbed for example by the desire for a cup of chai, then the Water element may have produced the desire for the pleasurable taste of it. Or the Fire element may have craved the self-confidence produced by the spicy herbs inside. Likewise, the Air element may have supported the particular desire for the sweet taste, to soothe some feeling of loneliness. Disidentification from these desires is always our choice, but the more we can keep the elements in our body balanced, the less energy we will need to spend on it.

Consequently, any yoga including *Jnana Yoga* is related to *Ayurveda*, the ancient vedic science of health[94]. The most important principle in *Ayurveda* directly regards the imbalances in the elements,

---

[94] See also 'Yoga & Ayurveda' on youtube.com/youyoga.

which are named *Doshas*[95]. The 'Doshas' both refer to temporary imbalances as to inborn imbalances that are regarded as body types. Imbalances in the Earth and Water elements lead to an excess or shortage of the Mucus *Dosha*[96] in the body. Imbalances in the Fire and Air elements lead to an excess or shortage of the Bile *Dosha*[97]. Imbalances in the Air and Space elements lead to an excess or shortage of the Wind *Dosha*[98] or gasses.

	Earth	Water	Fire	Air	Space
Mucus	x	x			
Bile			x	x	
Wind				x	x

Table 4. - Relationship between the Doshas and the Elements.

While these imbalances are the primary causes of most diseases of the physical body, they support and are themselves supported by emotional imbalances. Emotions may be triggered by any aspect of our being, yet the emotional feedback loop with the physical body will often determine the ease with which we can detach from any unpleasant feelings or attach to more agreeable emotions.

BILE	MUCUS	WIND
Anger	Sadness & Disgust	Fear

Table 5. - Emotional States supported by imbalanced Doshas.

---

[95] Sometimes 'Doshas' is translated as 'humors', but this refers to a somewhat similar ancient Greek system that is however limited to bodily fluids.

[96] The '*Kappha Dosha*'.

[97] The '*Pitta Dosha*'.

[98] The '*Vata Dosha*'.

More details on this subject originate in the ancient tantric science of *Rasa Sadhana*[99]. For example, if bile is in excess, anger is easily supported. If mucus is disturbed, sadness and disgust come easily. If wind is in excess, nervousness and anxiety will increase.

Furthermore, every individual body has an original body type or personal *Dosha* that can be defined as a particular mixture of the mucus, bile and wind *Dosha*s. People's inborn biochemistry can thus be dominated by either bile, mucus or wind, or by a combination of two of these or even have a relatively good balance between the three of them. In that way our body type defines the type of emotional imbalances that will be predominant in us, as well as the ways in which to balance ourselves in the elements.

Any imbalance in wind, mucus or bile will respectively create a disturbance in thinking, feeling or doing. For example, too many gasses in the intestines will irritate the nerves, so our thinking will become more nervous. Lack of *Prana* is the main opposite problem, decreasing our insight. Shortage of mucous may lead to 'dry' feelings and lack of empathy, while an excess of mucous may lead to becoming overly sensitive. When bile is low, not only will our digestive fire be weak, but we will also experience reduced confidence and increasing laziness. When bile is in excess, we may experience acid reflux, headaches, increased irritability and forceful actions.

To some degree, these imbalances can be directly detected by monitoring both our body temperature and the moisture in our mouth. Mucus is wet and cold, bile is hot and dry, while the gasses of the wind *Dosha* produce both a feeling of cold and dryness (see Table 6).

An uncomplicated way to work with the elements is for example to

---

[99] See 'The Yoga of the Nine Emotions: The Tantric Practice of Rasa Sadhana', Peter Marchand, Destiny Books 2006.

use some water and fresh ginger[100]. Excess in mucus can be easily reduced by increasing heat through taking some strong and hot ginger tea. Excess in bile can be reduced by increasing cold through the drinking of some water, best without added ice or the effect might be reversed. Excess in gasses must be tackled with a subtle combination of heat and moisture, using a milder, lukewarm ginger tea. If continuously observing ourselves includes keeping a watch over body temperature and tongue moisture, we can quickly discover any imbalances. Keeping just some water and fresh ginger nearby, can very often suffice to handle it. Of course, in case of more serious imbalances, seeking help from an Ayurvedic practitioner is advisable.

	BILE	MUCUS	WIND
TEMPERATURE	hot	cold	cold
MOISTURE	dry	moist	dry
INCREASE	strong tea	water	mild tea
DECREASE	water	strong tea	mild tea

Table 6. - Doshas, Temperature & Moisture
and how to change the Doshas by using either water or ginger tea.

Different foods are well known to produce more bile, mucus or wind, depending also on how they are prepared[101]. To satisfy the sense of taste so that no taste cravings disturb us, a meal should have all six primary tastes in proper proportions: sweet, sour, salty, pungent, bitter and astringent. Next to the direct effect of the taste, there is another more lasting impact during and after digestion. Many more details must be studied to balance the enormous impact digestion

---

[100] Compared to other hot spices that might also work, fresh ginger has the particular advantage of not being too much drying, which is especially useful when the gasses are imbalanced.

[101] See also 'Yoga Food' on youtube.com/youyoga.

has on our energy and emotional wellbeing[102].

Not only what we eat, but also how and when we eat is important. Avoiding overeating is a main way to combat negative emotions[103]. A very good practice here is to decide how much we will eat of a particular meal before our taste buds get involved. We fill our plate with what seems like the right amount of food and don't take second helpings.

Actual food fasts can be used to rebalance the elements and will strongly increase our capacity to hold mind still. We then become fully aware of the 'high' that our eating habits are all the time creating in our mind, muddling our focus. Meditation best happens before meals, and if for example during some holiday we would like to meditate a lot, then eating more sparingly is certainly advisable.

Physical exercise will aid digestion as well as the circulation of blood and other fluids in our body. Walking, running, yoga postures, etc. obviously help to remove excess stress from the body[104]. Grounding postures are especially needed to get 'out of our head' and connect to the Earth to release tension.

Particular postures are well known to promote mucus, bile or wind, or help to reduce them. Our daily yoga posture sequence should be created in accord with our personal *Dosha* or body type and adapted accordingly to any temporary imbalance in the elements – as shown in Table 7. For example, the famous sun salutation is very good (++) for daily practice in people dominated by mucus and also advisable for people dominated by the wind *Dosha* (+). However, those dominated by bile (-) would benefit much more from choosing the more cooling moon salutations for their everyday sequence (++).

Last but actually first, developing a comfortable sitting posture for

---

[102] See 'Ayurvedic Healing Cuisine', Harish Johari, Healing Arts Press 2000.

[103] In the words of Harish Johari 'better eat junk food than too much food'.

[104] See Chapter 7.

meditation is the original objective of all *Asana* posture practice, without which maintaining deep meditation is simply impossible[105].

	WIND	BILE	MUCUS
SITTING POSTURES			
Sidhasana (lotus)	++	+	+
Vajrasana (diamond)	++	+	+
Simhasana (lion)	+	-	++
Virasana (hero)	+		+
STANDING POSTURES			
Vrikshasana (tree)	++	++	
Trikonasana (triangle)	+	++	
Virabhadrasana (warrior)			+
INVERTED POSTURES			
Sirshasana (headstand)	+	-	+
Sarvangasana (schoulderstand)		+	+
Adho Mukha Vrksasana (handstand)			++
FORWARD BENDS			
Janu Sirshasana (head to knee)	++		-
Adho Mukha Svasana (downward dog)			+
Urdha Mukha Svasana (upward dog)			+
BACKWARD BENDS			
Bhujangaasana (cobra)	++	+	
Shalabhasana (locust)	++		+
Navasana (boat)		+	
Matsyasana (fish)		+	
Dhanurasana (bow)		+	+
Halasana (plough)			+
Ushtrasana (camel)			+
TWISTS			
Bharadvajasana (seated spinal twist)	+		
Padasana (noose twist)	+		
Ardha Matsyendrasana (lord of fishes)		+	
LYING POSES			
Balasana (fetus)	+	+	
Kurmasana (turtle)	+	++	
Yoga Mudra (yogic seal)	+	+	
Shavasana (corpse)	++	++	
SURYA NAMASKAR (sun salutation)	+	-	++
CHANDRA NAMASKAR (moon salutation)		++	-

Table 7. - Positive or Negative Impact of Daily Asana Practice.

---

[105] See Chapter 13.

So many other ways exist to balance any imbalance in the Space of our body, including many physical therapies such as massage, chiropractic manipulations, osteopathy, etc. Knowing some basic home remedies, with which to nip an imbalance in the bud, can be very helpful. It definitely beats letting the problem further aggravate, while we await a doctor's appointment. Last but not least, how we deal with sleep, sex and many other habits in life will also affect our elemental ability to go for peace, joy and love.

Physical wellbeing can of course not always be guaranteed, and then it is our choice to detach from any disturbing signals or not. Some yogic techniques will even consciously produce physical discomfort to teach us to distance ourselves from the body[106]. At all times, we should be aware of the transient nature of our body, which is why cremation grounds are often associated with profound yogic practice. We should never become obsessed with our food, exercise or other bodily comforts, lest that becomes a source of unhappiness, imbalance and untruth in itself. Healthy habits that meet our personal physical makeup are the best way to keep in balance[107]. As we grow older, the elements get out of control more easily, so it pays to develop those personal healthy habits while we are young. Yet, while a strict diet may sometimes be needed to restore balance, being too strict on food in the long run makes digestion too sensitive. It then becomes difficult to travel or otherwise having to eat less balanced foods.

The complementarity of things is so very much part of the way in which the nondual Self manifests within duality. Balancing the elements in our body is a very practical application of the law of unity in diversity, which is the law of love. Every element deserves some

---

[106] Especially *Sadhus* in India are known for their beds of nails or broken glass, as well as many other painful practices. One of them once told me it was a matter of creating some permanent discomfort, in order to never forget the true source of comfort.

[107] See Chapter 12.

attention, has some place within the whole, yet always in balance with the other elements. Giving each element its appropriate Space, will very much influence our feeling of love towards everyone and everything.

LOVE

Many of our love relationships are based upon a balanced exchange within the elements, even if also the more subtle energy bodies are very much involved[108]. We expect others to support and not threaten our elementary desires for security, pleasure, social status, connection, understanding and peace, that all relate to the elements[109]. However, misunderstandings can never be totally avoided, even if an attitude of open communication can resolve many of them.

If we keep the elements of our body in balance, then the related desires will be more balanced and so will our relationships be. For example, if we get distracted and forget to eat at the right time, both our bile and wind *Dosha*s will be disturbed by it. Dryness will be the result, which will irritate the nerves, further disturbing first the wind and then the bile. If then our beloved is just a little late in cooking dinner, the fire of our anger may be quickly ignited.

We are all children of the mother matter of Space and by extension of the elements. As such we are all kin, truly brothers and sisters. While being the same in basic consciousness and energy, we are also entirely unique, each one of us. Practicing unconditional love means that we accept everyone and everything as being in a particular place, in a specific state of body and mind, with specific natural needs and

---

[108] See Chapter 7.

[109] See Chapter 7.

desires.

While there is a tendency to measure others along our own scales, true love requires the empathy in seeing the other's point of view. While we have the duty to defend our own space, we can accept the same duty in others. Always dancing in harmony[110] with others and our environment is a much-overlooked part of the yogic path. However, nothing can disturb any real meditation as much as troubles within our relationships.

Love is a feeling and seeing of beauty. Seeing beauty, we create beauty. All arts are an expression of this realization. When we feel disturbed inside, beauty is hard to see and then art becomes therapy. From the peaceful silence of the Self, the entire universe is nothing but beautiful. This way, we see the beauty in every being we meet. When connecting to the inner beauty of another, the outer beauty becomes apparent, wrinkles included. To live life in love means to have the nature of a lotus flower. Roots deep into the mud, we shine brightly. The imperfect does not lessen the perfect. Others also having those roots does not reduce the radiance of the flowers they manifest.

Therefore, we connect, and sharing becomes the principal attitude when dealing with the matter of Space, which we anyhow receive from the same mother. While material wealth is always limited somehow, love and light, great cooking and heartfelt music can easily be shared without becoming less. Share simple living, high thinking, love.

Yet it is not so easy to love everyone, as the energies do not always match. It is natural to exercise our universal unconditional love first with one matching person in a love relationship[111]. If two people really love each other unconditionally, they will create a tremendous power.

---

[110] '*Dharma*', meaning 'harmony' or 'righteousness'.

[111] See also 'The Yoga of a Love Relationship' on youtube.com/youyoga.

They will be like a safe haven for each other, where they can always retreat, where they can ever find acceptance, comfort, gentleness and the Self. If two can find each other in such an unconditional bubble of love, this bubble may expand and influence other people, maybe the children, family, friends, the neighborhood, etc. It is how a loving community is often created in practice.

The divine Self is present in everyone. We do not need to love the people on Mars, as the Self is also there taking care of the love they need. We start with those close by - that is the natural way. Of course, the ego can and will make a mess of it sometimes, but that will always be the case, whether we love one or everyone. Do not let any ideas on celibacy stand in the way of a heartfelt desire to connect with someone special. If we all become renunciates, then where will the ones get born who truly feel the effortless need to renounce?

7

TIME

The primary energy of time that emerged from the unchanging bliss or *Ananda* aspect of the Self, is eternally changing, dancing, pulsating, breathing. It is the very power of illusion and playfulness[112]. This mysterious 'electromagnetic' energy named *Prana* takes on so many forms, from the very first spark of the Big Bang to the vibrations found within the tiniest of subatomic particles, the energy of moonlight, the life force within the air that we breathe, the mental energy of anxiety, the pure bliss of the Self, etc. Ever changing, ever confusing, ever playing for the very sake of the play, of life itself.

Change cannot exist without duality as it always creates a duality between two opposite states in time. Something hot getting cold, someone peaceful becoming stressed, some this turning into that. Given this ever changing, intrinsically dual nature of the life force, the yoke of yoga[113] is not just symbolizing union, but also balancing. When plus and minus are brought in balance, the result is zero, neutrality, nonduality. Likewise working with the life force means to create a neutral, nondual energy by balancing opposing energies, whether they come as dualities, trinities or in even higher diversity.

Fortunately, we live in a cosmos, not in total chaos. Behind the dazzling multitude of phenomena created by the power of Time and the life force, we can discover the more essential changes taking

---

[112] That power appears as the cosmic illusion (*Maya*) and as the divine play (*Leela*).

[113] Yoga refers to the root word 'yoke', a wooden bar one carries on both shoulders to unite and balance two opposite objects, such as buckets.

57

place and learn to work with them. To that purpose, yogic science offers us many ways to better comprehend the nature of our vital energy. So, fasten your seatbelt, as this really long chapter will guide us through the many games that our *Prana* plays, and how we can play along with it.

As consciousness and energy are just two sides of the same beingness, some teachings[114] equate *Prana* with the Self. It is somewhat confusing because *Prana* is usually seen as the energy that we absorb through breathing. Practices related to *Prana* are mostly breathing exercises. Yet surely, with every breath we take, we inhale consciousness as well as *Prana*. The particular *Prana* in manifestation that most directly relates to consciousness is actually *Kundalini*, which we will explore at the end of this chapter.

Eternal Time is of course a great object of meditation, as already explained in Chapter 3 as a seed-based practice. Moreover, time as the eternal life force brings us the truth of immortality. As we will explore at length in Chapter 8, our souls are eternal and death is the illusion. Time is the tree that sheds its leaves in autumn only to make space for new fresh leaves to be born in spring. The energy of Time is the great mother of all and teaches us to love the impermanence of things. Eternal time teaches non attachment to whatever comes, as it always has to go at some time to make room for something else.

THE PRANIC BODY

The first subtle body that exists within and around the physical body is the *Pranic* body[115], where we directly experience our gross

---

[114] 'Consciousness and the Absolute: The Final Talks of Sri Nisargadatta Maharaj', edited by Jean Dunn, The Acorn Press.

[115] '*Pranamayi Kosha*', the 'body of vital energy'.

feelings such as anger or joy. It is to be seen as the interface between body and mind, affecting both and being affected by both. Truly all subtle bodies are made of *Prana*, but in the *Pranic* body not much else is there but pure energetic vibration that produces the sensation of particular emotions. It is commonly called the *Aura*, and if we meet someone and enter his or her energy field, we can feel it affecting our own energy. The *Pranic* body extends to about an arm length from the physical body. Keeping two arm lengths distance helps when we do not want someone's gross energy to affect us so directly. This may be especially advisable when dealing with emotionally unstable people.

As the *Pranic* life force is ever fluctuating, the *Pranic* body continuously creates changes in our mind. As our primary source of *Prana* is breath, breathing patterns strongly influence the quality of our mental activity. Moreover, because of the brain, mind needs a continuous supply of *Prana* through breath, otherwise it ultimately has to stop thinking.

'Stop breath and mind will stop' is one of the most essential yogic insights, teaching us how to slow down thoughts or stop thinking altogether. Breath retention[116] is one of the most powerful breathing practices, as it immediately calms the *Pranic* body. It allows one to quite instantly reduce any unpleasant mental activity and reconnect to the Self. Moreover, it is a fabulous aid in meditation.

It is advisable to hold the breath after inhaling for as long as it feels comfortable, followed by a long exhale. To hold the breath after the exhale is also possible, but it should not be done for very long without proper training. Ultimately the practice of breath retention involves the total cessation of breath in deep meditation. While anyone can

---

[116] '*Kumbhaka*', referring to the torso as a 'pot' filled in this case with air.

practice mild forms of breath retention without much further information, advanced breath retention practices require proper teaching. There is the use of particular 'locks' within the physical body[117], and the correct buildup of proportions between the times taken for inhaling, retention and exhaling[118].

NINE EMOTIONAL ENERGIES

The nine *Rasas*[119] are the essential energies of the *Pranic* body, that represent a set of emotions and moods that belong to the same 'family' of emotions. While the nine *Rasas* themselves are clearly defined energies affecting body and mind, the resulting emotions[120] manifest in a multitude of varieties. Their interpretation is affected by personal and cultural backgrounds.

RASA	RELATED EMOTIONS & EXPRESSIONS
Love	Beauty, aesthetic sentiment, devotion
Humor	Joy, laughter, sarcasm
Wonder	Curiosity, astonishment, mystery
Calmness	Peace, relaxation, rest.
Anger	Violence, irritation, stress
Courage	Heroism, determination, confidence
Sadness	Compassion, pity, sympathy
Fear	Terror, anxiety, nervousness, worry
Disgust	Depression, dissatisfaction, self-pity

Table 8. – The Nine Rasas or Emotional Essences

---

[117] Named '*Bandhas*', meaning 'to hold'.

[118] Most teachings will culminate in the 1-4-2 proportion representing the times for inhaling, retention and exhaling, but many other systems exist.

[119] 'The Yoga of the Nine Emotions: The Tantric Practice of Rasa Sadhana', Peter Marchand, Destiny Books 2006.

[120] '*Bhavas*' or emotions.

Knowing the particular mechanisms of each of the nine *Rasas* helps us to see why a certain mood comes and stays. We can use that knowledge to achieve more emotional control. We can also utilize our emotions as masks, which we can put on if needed in communication. Some people for example may not be able to take a simple 'no' seriously, if we do not perform a little show of anger.

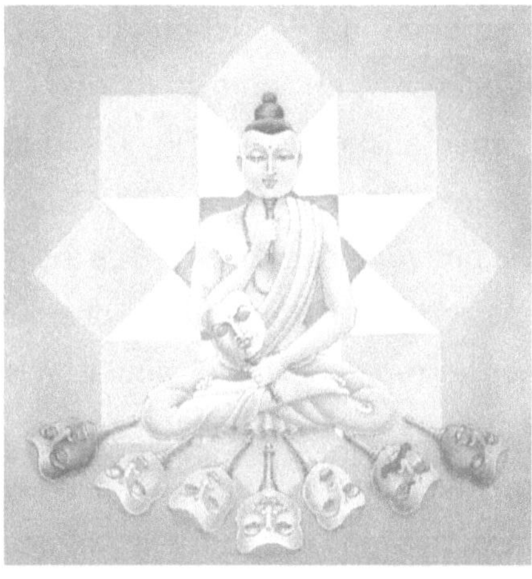

ill. 14. - The 9 Rasas as masks used by the Yogi[121].

These emotional essences are recognized by everyone and most cultures, yet most people know little about them. The yogic traditions offer great insight into their relationship to other Pranic energies. The *Rasas* can be particularly helpful in realizing the principal objective of yoga: to be happy whenever we want. In Chapter 6 we have already discussed how the elements of the physical body affect them, and in the following paragraphs, we will encounter them very often when particular manifestations of *Prana* influence them.

---

[121] Painting by Pieter Weltevrede.

Of course, the attachments of the ego are the principal cause of all unpleasant emotions. There the subconscious is revealed as the most fundamental origin of these feelings, containing the most powerful emotional triggers[122]. Learning how to play with their energetic nature makes it a lot easier to stay away from unhappy feelings, yet it is still our not-so-conscious choice to attach or not.

The emotional essences are principally differentiated by the way in which we experience our attachments. Anger comes when someone else has disrespected some attachment. Fear comes when our attachment seems threatened in the future, whether by somebody else, nature, ourselves or whatever. Sadness comes when an attachment is already gone, which causes the pain of separation. Disgust and depression come when some attachment is gone and we blame ourselves. All represent the essential error made by the ego to strongly attach to something, while by nature all things have to go sometime. The ego has often such fixed ideas on what it needs to be happy, that it prefers unhappiness to the joy of letting go what goes and seeing what is next.

Agreeable emotions represent more truthful ways in dealing with attachment. The very nature of love is to attach, yet we can at the same time be detached from that attachment. We just accept that the time for detachment will come and we can even embrace the natural pain that it may bring. If some attachment goes or is threatened, we can laugh about it, feeling humor in seeing the joke that is the ego. Does not every detachment open space for some new attachment or love? Or we may feel wonder at the miracle through which attachments seem to come and go in life. We can muster the courage to keep on working for our attachments, even if we know that they are

---

[122] See Chapter 8.

temporary. Peace then is the *Rasa* without *Rasa*, an emotion that is not very emotional, neutral, which is created by accepting detachment.

Rasa Sadhana is an ancient tantric tradition of emotional fasting[123]. We promise ourselves that for some time we will not get involved with one of the less agreeable *Rasas* or will fully focus on one of the more agreeable *Rasas*[124]. When doing this practice with anger for example, whenever some irritation comes, we just remember our promise not to give in to it. That will create a distance between ourselves and the angry feeling, which is often sufficient to dissolve the anger. If not, so many other more energetic techniques can be used to help dissolve it, such as breath, diet, *mantra*, etc. This is not about emotional suppression of course, rather about exercising ourselves in letting feelings go. Through such regular exercise, we learn that we can really master our emotions. After some time, that may happen quite effortlessly, even if sometimes a deeper feeling related to a more profound attachment may first need to be thoroughly felt, before it can be dissolved[125].

THE MOVEMENT OF PRANA

Distinct types of Pranic energy can also be found in the way that *Prana* moves within the body through the intermediate of the Air element[126] :

---

[123] 'The Yoga of the Nine Emotions: The Tantric Practice of Rasa Sadhana', Peter Marchand, Destiny Books 2006.

[124] We usually start with one day, then extending that to a few days, always with some time in between. This can be slowly increased to a week, a month, a year, ...

[125] See Chapter 8, in 'The Dark Night of the Soul'.

[126] Because of this relationship between *Prana* and the Air element, the 5 *Pranas* are often named the 5 '*Vayus*' or Airs.

- Basic *Prana* we find where it enters the body, making an inward movement, like in breathing of course, but also through the senses, food, water, etc. It directly provides energy to the brain and is the source of all other forms of *Prana*.

- *Apana* represents the opposite movement of energy, leaving the body through the exhale and in urination, defecation, menstruation, etc. *Apana* is usually the most impure, polluted form of *Prana*, which is why it is outgoing[127].

- *Vyana* is the *Prana* that expands into the entire body, circulating vital energy along with nutrients, oxygen, etc. The primary center of *Vyana* is the area of lungs and heart.

- *Udana* is the life force that is being used to do all kinds of things, like moving, speaking, growing... It is associated with the throat area, dominating our will power.

- *Samana* is a churning, 'cooking' form of *Prana*, centered around the navel. It digests food, water and air, as well as all kinds of mental impressions.

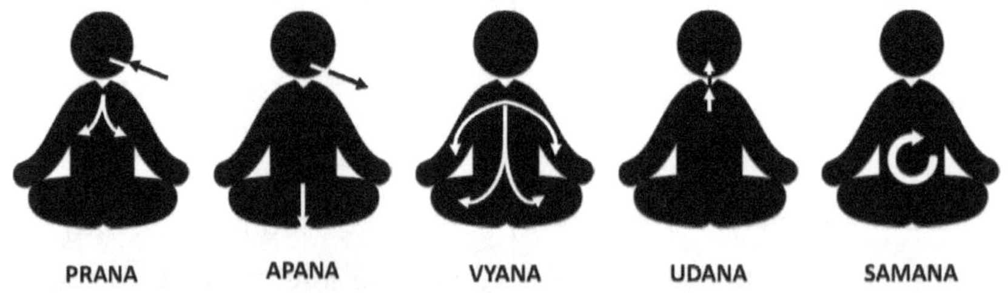

ill. 15. - Primary Movements of Prana.

If one of these movements of *Prana* becomes disturbed, the others will soon be affected. Any such disturbance will rapidly unbalance all

---

[127] Ejaculation and childbirth are also outgoing functions of *Apana*, though obviously for other reasons than 'impurity'.

elements of the physical body as well. Through the Wind *Dosha*, these *Pranas* are responsible for all functional movements of the elements within the physical body, as Bile and Mucus do not move by themselves. Disturbed *Prana* will unbalance the *Doshas*, which will not only impact our health, but also our mental stability and ability to concentrate and meditate.

Getting to know the different movements of *Prana* and learning to master them is a broad subject. As *Prana* always follows our attention wherever we concentrate in the body, visualization is a major technique to make the energy flow in the right way. Pranic healing[128] principally uses the same method through the contact between two Pranic bodies.

While the many yoga poses help to keep the physical body healthy and flexible, their impact on the Pranic body should not be underestimated. In steadying a pose while holding the breath after an inhale, blocked energies in the gross energy body may be freed from various parts of the body. They can then be released into the Earth upon the exhale and the release of the posture. Especially as long as a practitioner still experiences occasional emotional imbalances, physical exercise is advised to prevent such blockages from influencing the more subtle levels of our being. To consciously remove them means to prevent them from reemerging whenever we try to relax.

Keeping *Apana* from polluting the other *Pranas* is perhaps the most essential practice related to the five *Pranas*, which is when regular bowel movements suddenly get high spiritual relevance[129]. Especially before sunrise, when the gravity of the sun naturally

---

[128] Mostly recognized these days as the Japanese tradition of '*Reiki*', *Pranic* healing is also well known within the science of *Ayurveda*.

[129] See 'Dhanwantari' by Harish Johari, Rupa Publications India 2001.

separates *Prana* from *Apana*[130], first eliminating stool and urine is particularly balancing and purifying. The seated warrior pose with emphasis on the hollow lower back can be very helpful to practice just before going to the bathroom, whenever bowel movements are blocked. Starting any yoga or meditation practice with a few deep sighs clears any residual *Apana* from the lungs, attached to the waste product carbon dioxide.

THE VIBRATION OF PRANA

The three *Guna*s are modes of energy vibration in the life force, independent of where and how *Prana* is moving in the body. They are present everywhere in the universe and help us to see the fundamental dynamics of change. Basically, some energy is 'not' vibrating and unchanging, some energy is strongly vibrating and changing, and some energy is gently vibrating, beyond changing or unchanging.

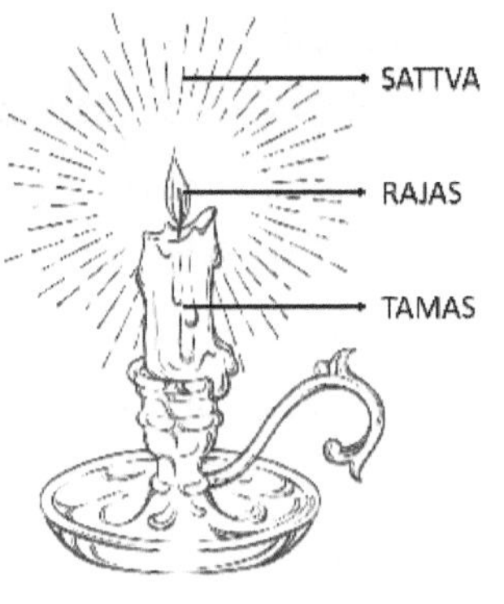

ill. 16. - The Gunas of the Candle.

This way the hard unchanging wax of a candle is called *Tamasic*, the ever-changing flame is *Rajasic* and the light of the candle is *Sattvic*, which is the essence or purpose of the candle. *Tamasic* energy is pure potentiality, inactive, dark, dense and unchanging. *Rajasic* energy is pure manifestation, active, comes in many colors and densities and is ever changing. The *Sattvic* energy, which is the closest in feeling to the bliss of the Self, is the

---

[130] See Chapter 12.

manifestation of the unmanifested essence, neither active nor inactive, light, vibrating yet unchanging, the most essential of all *Guna*s. Flowers are among the most *Sattvic* things in the universe. The *Gunas* are so important in *Tantric Advaita* that I have chosen them for the cover image of this book. Within the teaching lineage of my healing work, white represents *Sattva*, yellow *Rajas* and red *Tamas*. It basically means that every energy is invited to join the healing ritual, independent of their *Guna*.

As consciousness and energy are ever intertwined, the *Guna*s also represent different levels of understanding. When our energy is dark, *Tamasic*, then ignorance and negative thinking usually prevail. When we are filled with the multicolored *Rajasic* energy, ignorance is still rather present, but aimed at applying our understanding, trying to create a change for the better. When we enjoy the bliss of the *Sattvic* energy, which is full of light, wisdom comes easily.

From the bliss of the Self, manifestation emerged as pure *Prana* with a *Sattvic* energy vibration. As the universe expanded and changed, that same energy became *Rajasic*. When the *Rajasic* changes started interacting with each other, a kind of friction or inertia was the result, which created the *Tamasic* energy of the denser manifestation of the universe. Human spiritual evolution means to return to the bliss of the source, reconverting the *Tamasic* energy back into the *Sattvic* energy, through the intermediate of the *Rajasic* energy of the action that we may call yoga.

Here we find an especially important insight from the vedic seers, which in a way clarifies the main narrative of this book. To produce light from the candle, whose potential is hidden in the dormant energy of the wax, we need to burn the candle. Some action is needed to reach that subtle vibration which is beyond action or inaction. To move from *Tamas* to *Sattva*, more often than not *Rajas* is needed, energetic transformation is needed, effort is needed. If this power of change is properly trained and used, not much of it is actually required.

Very often spiritual people when feeling unhappy while being low in energy, try to find solace in directly going for the silence and bliss of the Self. The chance that this works is rather slim, depending on practice and the level of personal growth. Some action, some movement, some transformation of the energy may be required. If then first we use different postures, breathing techniques, concentration exercises, etc. the *Tamasic* energy will be activated into *Rajasic* energy. Once the energy is *Rajasic*, we will literally have the power of change at hand to harmonize the level of activity, ending up in the silence and bliss of *Sattva*.

In life it is only natural to encounter *Tamas*, *Rajas* and *Sattva*. To live means to move, which is the *Rajasic* energy. Movement consumes energy, so then rest is needed, sleep is needed, which is *Tamasic* in nature. And even if we are unaware of it, the *Sattvic* energy is always in our presence, inspired by the bliss of the Self. Likewise, we cannot say that a person is 100% *Tamasic*. Maybe the *Tamasic* energy will rather dominate, but some *Rajasic* energy will also be there, and even *Sattva* will always be present somehow. Other people may be very *Sattvic* in nature, but some more *Rajasic* work will always be needed, naturally followed by some more *Tamas*. Especially rare are those who can maintain a purely *Sattvic* energy even while acting, so that also no more *Tamas* in terms of sleep is needed.

While we can say that the *Sattvic* energy is the closest to the truth, the closest to the bliss of the Self, it is not the truth. The trinity of the *Gunas* is truly the one nondual energy of the life force, just as ice, water and water vapor are all forms of H_2O. *Prana* is eternally omnipresent within manifestation and its ever-fluctuating vibrational nature is expressed by the *Gunas*. Within the final stages of spiritual growth, through the deepest states of meditation, any attachment to any of these primary modes of energy including *Sattva* must be dissolved[131]. So, if we feel tired, we rest. If we feel lots of energy, we act. And if our energy feels rather balanced, we enjoy the bliss but do not overly attach to it. If we can balance *Rajas* and *Tamas*, giving each their proper time and place, the neutral *Sattvic* energy will always be readily available.

There is nothing wrong with the *Tamasic* desire to sleep, but if *Tamas* is too dominant in a person, that desire will come at the wrong time. It then leads to useless activities that cannot truly be enjoyed because of the state of low energy. There is nothing wrong with the *Rajasic* desire to talk, but if *Rajas* is too dominant in the mind, the resulting chatter will only get on other people's nerves. And there is nothing wrong in desiring the bliss of *Sattva*, but if an excess of *Sattva* is there at the wrong time, some natural work coming our way may not get done. As these desires can be fulfilled or not, they produce our very basic emotions. To avoid unhappy feelings resulting from friction between the *Gunas*, remember that everything has a right time.

The emotional essences or *Rasas* of sadness, fear and depression are *Tamasic* in nature. While sometimes they may lead to lots of mental activity, they produce inaction or actions that are unproductive. Love, joy, wonder, courage and anger are *Rajasic* in nature. They readily bring desires for action, which may be fruitful or not. Only the *Rasa* of peace is truly *Sattvic*, but as this somewhat special emotional essence can be mixed with other emotional

---

[131] Patanjali Yoga Sutras 3.51.

essences[132], it can make them more *Sattvic* too.

TAMAS	RAJAS	SATTVA
Sadness	Love	Peace
Fear	Joy	
Disgust	Wonder	
	Courage	
	Anger	

Table 9. - Relationship between Rasas & Gunas.

The *Guna*s are primary promotors of particular desires, when their energy interacts with the five elements of our body, and consciousness identifies with it. When *Tamasic* energy dominates, one's desires usually do not move beyond those of Earth (security) and Water (pleasure). When the energy is more *Rajasic*, the desires of Fire (status), Air (love) and Space (understanding) come into play. When we are in a *Sattvic* mood, desires are generally lightened and tend towards moving beyond the elements into more contemplative or meditative states.

Proper food and digestion are among the main ways in which to avoid unnecessary and unfruitful *Tamasic* or *Rajasic* energy in our lives. In any case, some more *Tamasic* foods such as pulses are needed as storehouses of gross energy, but they are usually harder to digest and easily produce a dull feeling. *Rajasic* foods such as refined sugars bring energy more directly and are easily digestible, but they may be over stimulating. Overuse may lead to excessive and

---

[132] The other *Rasas* cannot be mixed, even though one might fluctuate rapidly from one to another, such as in the state of jealousy, which involves both anger and fear, but not really simultaneously.

exhausting mental and/or physical activity, which is rapidly followed by *Tamasic* heaviness instead of *Sattvic* lightness. The most *Sattvic* foods are fresh fruits, the favorite food of saints.

Generally speaking, fresh foods are to be preferred over old, canned or frozen foods, which are highly *Tamasic*. Highly refined *Rajasic* foods such as sugar and of course also stimulants like coffee are best moderated if we want our meditation practice to be somewhat peaceful. Balanced cooking also means that while heating reduces the need for digestion in *Tamasic* foods, the same 'pre-digestive' heat must be applied gently in cooking to preserve the more subtle *Sattvic* foods. Herbs and spices give food a more *Sattvic* nature and some are particularly helpful to stimulate the digestive system, so that it produces less dullness. The proportion in which we mix *Tamasic*, *Rajasic* and *Sattvic* foods in our diet is quite personal and dependent on the kind of activities that we are involved with at any given time. The art of spiritual cooking combines the knowledge of the *Dosha*s with that of the *Guna*s. There is much more to learn here, but that goes quite beyond the scope of this book[133].

Physical exercise should always happen following the *Guna*s. When the body feels tired and rigid, and the mind is rather dull while it is not the right time for sleep, then more active physical exercise is needed to remove the inertia. When the body feels nervous, and the mind too excited, milder physical exercise followed by the action of conscious relaxation are logical to generate the alert calmness required for meditation. Grounding is another essential yogic practice, such as in the corpse pose[134]. The use of *Prana* visualization can be particularly effective to release any excess energy into Mother Earth.

---

[133] See 'Ayurvedic Healing Cuisine', Harish Johari, Healing Arts Press 2000.

[134] See also the 'Extended Corpse Pose' video on youtube.com/youyoga.

Spiritual progress is not about flying, it's about growing upwards into higher consciousness like a tree into the sky, firmly rooted.

Last but obviously not least, breath is a major way in which to control the *Guna*s and rapidly change them as needed. *Tamasic* breathing is slow and shallow. *Rajasic* breathing is fast and deep or shallow. *Sattvic* breathing is slow and deep. When we want to move from *Tamas* to *Sattva*, breathing more deeply may work. If not, then first some faster and deeper *Rajasic* breathing is needed. To move from *Rajas* to *Sattva*, we slow down breath, but keep it rather deep.

TAMAS	RAJAS	SATTVA
Slow & Shallow	Fast & Deep or Shallow	Slow & Deep

Table 10. - Relationship between Gunas & Breath.

THE STORAGE OF PRANA

Prana, *Tejas* and *Ojas* represent the different forms of *Prana* as they are found within our more subtle bodies. *Ojas* is a storehouse of *Prana* and *Tejas* the fiery energy that is produced through the liberation of *Prana* from *Ojas*. *Prana* here means the life force that we inhale through breathing and serves the immediate energetic or electromagnetic needs of our being, especially those of the nerves and the brain. It most directly relates to the element of air in the body.

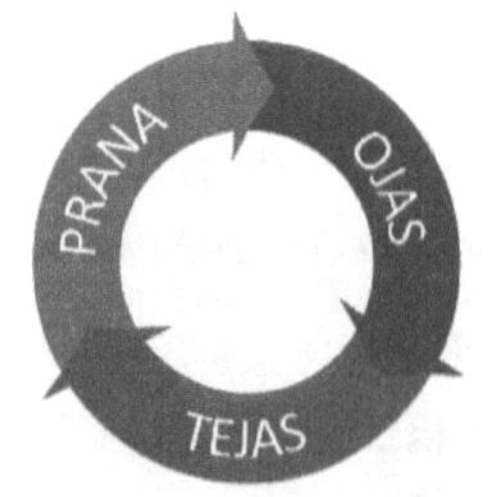

ill. 17. - Relationship between Prana, Tejas & Ojas.

Tejas is a form of *Prana* that is related to the fire element. Just as the fire element aids in the digestion of foods, *Tejas* aids in the digestion of impressions, feelings and thoughts. It is the light or power of intuitive seeing, which is a knowing. While *Prana* promotes the more usual thinking, spiritual understanding and intuitive insights very much depend on the availability of *Tejas*.

Ojas is a more condensed, 'oily' form of *Pranic* energy related to the water element. Yet, it remains subtle, purely energetic, and not physical. If it was physical and we could bottle it, it would be an elixir of life[135]. It is a *Pranic* energy reserve that provides both physical and mental/emotional endurance, healing, nourishment, self-confidence and the capacity to love.

Whatever *Prana* is absorbed through breath without being needed, our energy system will convert it to *Ojas* for later use. From *Ojas*, *Tejas* can be created, and from *Tejas*, *Prana* can be regenerated. Young people naturally have an abundance of *Ojas*, but as we get older this natural lubricating 'radiance' gets more easily depleted. To conserve *Ojas* is quite essential for maintaining good health, while it also determines how long we can stay in the deeper meditative stages. When breath in deep meditation is very much slowed down or even entirely suspended[136], then *Prana* will be generated from *Ojas* through *Tejas*. Our *Ojas* reserve will then determine how much time we get before our body will take us out of the trance state due to lack of *Prana*.

To some degree, *Prana*, *Tejas* and *Ojas* are directly affected by the imbalances called *Doshas* in the physical body. Taking good care of

---

[135] Also known as '*Amrit*'.

[136] See Chapter 13.

the elements in our body[137] is a primary way in which to economize our life force. That will very much determine whether we will have the energy or power to do what we want to do, whether we want to set up a business or aspire for deeper meditation. It will particularly impact our natural immunity, the endocrine system, digestion, fertility, the nervous system, etc.

The preservation of *Ojas* is a broad subject, which may involve diet, herbs and spices, emotional balance, control of sensory and sexual energy, as well as of course breathing. The habit of deep breathing builds *Ojas*, especially through long exhales. The feeling of love and devotion equally creates *Ojas*.

THE POLARITY OF PRANA

While the *Gunas* represent the changing or unchanging vibration of the life force, *Rajasic* changes within the life force are understood as a matter of polarity. The electromagnetic nature of the life force pulsates essentially in the same way as electricity does in a wire between a positive pole and a negative pole. One pole releases energy, while the other pole absorbs it. Both poles are essential for this movement to happen. In yogic science, the basic polarity within the life force is expressed as the fluctuation of solar and lunar energies, which are entirely complementary. One is fully dependent on the other for change to be possible. They are found at work within the smallest particles and the largest galaxies, as well as within ourselves. Truly, they are the one energy of change that is the Pranic life force.

The solar energy is electrical, acidic, heating and extrovert in

---

[137] See Chapter 6.

nature. It is active, verbal, rational, organizing and creating. The lunar energy is magnetic, alkaline, cooling and introvert in nature. It is passive, visual, emotional, caring and healing. Solar energy is seen as male and lunar energy as female, because generally the solar energy is more dominant in men and the lunar energy is more dominant in women. Yet we all have both these energies that are vital for life and some women are more solar than some men, and vice versa[138].

The recognition of this basic polarity may provide some insight and a little more peace into the typical discussions between men and women. It makes it clear how our largely patriarchal society tends to promote solar over lunar energies, rationality over emotion, suppressing emotions as a means to control them. It explains many of the problems in modern society, as well as within ourselves.

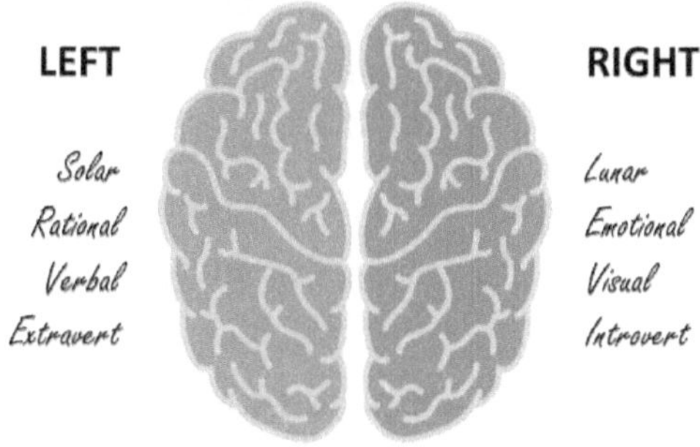

ill. 18. - Solar & Lunar Thinking in the Brain.

Solar and lunar polarity can be directly experienced within our internal dialogues. Very often this dialogue is dominated by some disagreement between thinking and feeling, which may be expressed as our 'head' not agreeing with our 'heart'. While indeed 'head and

---

[138] Everyone has the right to be as solar or lunar as they want to be.

heart' relates to thinking and feeling, this polarity is also present within the twin hemispheres of our brain. Thinking in the left hemisphere is more solar and rational, while in the right hemisphere it is more lunar and emotional. To stop thinking in meditation, the dialogue between both sides must be overcome. On the energetic level it means to balance solar and lunar energies into a more neutral energy.

This objective brings us to the rather fundamental question why does our nose have two nostrils? We have two eyes to see in three dimensions and two ears to locate the source of sounds. If it takes two to tango, why not have two mouths? Quite recently, Western science also came up with the answer, which anyone can easily observe within themselves. When we strongly inhale through the nose, usually one nostril feels cooler because it is more open than the other. Only sometimes we may experience that both nostrils are equally open, which is the moment when dominance changes, which takes about 10 breaths. This ever-fluctuating nostril dominance in fact continuously alternates dominance between the two brain hemispheres, between emotional and rational thinking. On average during the daytime, nostril and thus brain hemisphere dominance will change about every 1 to 2 hours.

It has also been observed by Western science that when the left nostril is dominant, the right hemisphere is more active, resulting in more visual and emotional thinking. When the right nostril is dominant, the left hemisphere is more active, resulting in more auditive and rational thinking. When one nostril is more dominant, the corresponding olfactory nerve is more cooled down by the incoming airflow[139]. As a result, the brain hemisphere on the same side becomes less active, giving dominance to the brain hemisphere on

---

[139] More recent research also points to the importance of the ionic stimulation of nerves.

the opposite side.

This extraordinary system is supposed to be more successful in evolutionary theory, as only lunar or only solar thinking leads to lower adaptability. Just as the movement of electrical currents requires positive and negative poles, alternating solar and lunar thinking is needed for our thinking to move ahead or evolve more rapidly. Evolution did not however consider how confusing this brain polarity can be[140], nor that it makes meditation a lot more difficult.

Alternate nostril breathing[141] is the yogic answer to this problem. When we want to be really silent inside, a few minutes of alternate nostril breathing can make it easier. If continued, the reduced activity in the brain will bring a naturally sustained balance between both hemispheres and both nostrils. Alternate nostril breathing usually means we start inhaling through the left nostril, and then exhale through the right nostril. Then we inverse the exercise by inhaling through the right nostril and exhaling through the left, and so on. The nostrils can be blocked using the tip of the thumb or a special hand posture[142].

Lunar breathing is more suitable for relaxation and actual meditation, while solar breathing helps with concentration. It means we can adapt nostril dominance according to the phase of meditation we find ourselves in. If for example concentration some day is really hard, block the left nostril while continuing the practice until the concentration becomes stable.

At sunset and sunrise, when the solar daytime changes to the lunar nighttime and vice versa, both nostrils become equally

---

[140] Ask those stigmatized as 'bipolar' by psychiatrists, while we are all 'bipolar' to some degree.

[141] *'Nadi Shodana'*; the 'purification' of the 'channels'.

[142] *'Nadi Shodana Mudra'*.

dominant for a while, and meditation is a lot easier. As lunar energy is generally more suitable for meditation, meditating during the night will work much better than during the day, while sunrise remains best. Adapting one's activities to the natural rhythms of sun and moon is another major aspect of balancing solar and lunar energies[143].

Solar and lunar breathing also correlate with bringing heat or cold in the body, producing respectively a more acidic or more alkaline blood chemistry. This is highly relevant for health and particularly in balancing the elements and related desires. Here we find special breathing techniques that are particularly cooling[144] or heating[145].

Whenever some imbalance in the elements manifests as a physical or mental/emotional problem, one can stop it by immediately changing the dominant nostril. Different methods exist, such as lying down on the opposite side of the body for a few minutes, using a pressure point just below the armpit on the same side as the dominant nostril[146] or putting a cotton ball plug in one nostril.

To consciously adapt nostril dominance by will power alone to whatever activity one undertakes, as well as to the astronomical solar and lunar energy patterns, is known as the science of *Swar Yoga*[147]. Left and right nostril breathing also affect dominance of the same sides of the body, which is the entrance into *Hatha Yoga* practice, even if that tradition goes quite beyond[148].

---

[143] '*See Chapter 12.*

[144] Mainly '*Shitali*' and '*Shitkari*'.

[145] Mainly '*Ujjayi*' and '*Kapalabhati*'.

[146] Pressure point at the 5th intercostal, a few inches below the armpit, easily affected by putting the hand in the armpit and pressing on it with the arm.

[147] See 'Breath, Mind, and Consciousness', by Harish Johari, Destiny Books 1989.

[148] 'There seems to be a lot of discussion whether '*Ha*' and '*Tha*' really refer to sun and moon.

PRANA & DESIRE

The importance of solar and lunar energies is not limited to the brain or the mental body. They equally alternate within our more subtle bodies and thus within the subtle energy currents or channels known as *Nadis*. Out of the total of 72,000 *Nadis* said to be present in our system, the three most important ones are the lunar, the solar and the neutral *Nadi*[149].

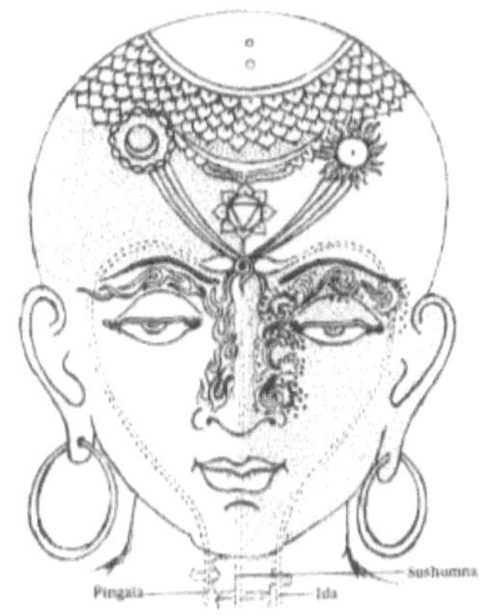

ill. 19. - Relationship between Nostrils, main Nadis and our Brain[150].

In left nostril breathing, the lunar channel is activated, and in right nostril breathing the solar channel. When both nostrils are in balance, the neutral channel becomes active, which plays a vital role in the energetic process of meditation, as well as within spiritual growth. It immediately stops that endless doubting created by alternating solar and lunar thinking, bringing the certainty of nondual knowing.

Spiritual growth can be seen as the natural maturing of our desires through the 5 elements of our body[151]. This primarily happens within the energy centers of the *Chakras*, which are predominantly solar or lunar. While all *Chakras* have solar and lunar energy, the first, third and fifth *Chakras* are predominantly solar and relate more to thinking, expression and acting. The second, fourth and sixth *Chakras* are

---

[149] Respectively, the '*Ida, Pingala & Sushumna Nadis*'.

[150] Using fire to symbolize solar energy and water for lunar energy.

[151] See also Chapter 8.

predominantly lunar and relate more to feeling, impression and enjoying. In 7th *Chakra* the neutral energy dominates, but when that stage is reached that will also be the case in the other *Chakra*s.

To overcome the blockages in one of the *Chakra*s means to balance the lunar and solar energies at work there. When the solar energy is too dominant for example in the first *Chakra* in relation to work and money, it leads to workaholism, unhealthy expectations, greedily disregarding the needs of others, etc. When the lunar energy is too dominant in this *Chakra*, the work may suffer from a lack in clear confidence, objectives and planning.

Likewise, one might say that industrial agriculture is far too solar to sustainably work with soil and nature. Organic agriculture is more lunar and keeps natural balances intact. We may discuss endlessly about all of this, and that is also part of life. A culture that knows how to balance solar and lunar energies, will be much more capable of harmoniously dealing with all its issues. It may start with teaching kids alternate nostril breathing.

To only focus on the truth of pure awareness and disregard whatever we feel, suppressing an energy that really does not feel good, is actually a very rational, solar, 'male' approach. To be so impressed by whatever we feel that the very idea of distancing from it seems ludicrous, is the very emotional, lunar, 'female' approach. The more balanced, neutral approach is to detach from whatever unhappy feeling comes, accept it for what it is and simultaneously change it for the better.

Accepting that a feeling exists does not mean that we cannot try to change it. Trying to change it does not mean that we do not accept it. As the nature of the energy is to always change anyhow, why not play along? Many people feel that they have to resist something in order to change it, but one should see beyond this duality the wisdom in the complementarity of accepting and changing things. Suppose we feel some anger that seems out of place, but is hard to forget about. Then we first observe the anger without judging it, accept ourselves in having that anger, rather than be dissatisfied with ourselves for being affected by it. Only then we may be able to let it go. If we simply resist it by pushing it away, it will revisit us later.

Balancing our desires by balancing our *Pranic* energy is a main way to achieve the basic peace that is required to enter deep meditation. Then the very miraculous work of unifying consciousness and energy can ultimately happen.

THE PRANA OF CONSCIOUSNESS

Consciousness and energy are one beingness, yet in manifestation they are in a way also separated. The essence of the essence of the purest, nondual *Pranic* energy is known as the *Kundalini* energy. It is coiled like a spring or a snake in the first chakra, while consciousness naturally resides in a *Chakra* located within the heart *Chakra*[152]. In meditation withdrawing inside means that consciousness moves into the so-called *corpus callosum*, a neutral 'space' that connects the lunar and solar brain hemispheres, traditionally named the cave of the bumble bee[153]. Through practice, the *Kundalini* energy can move upwards, piercing the *Chakra*s and finally unite with consciousness in that 'cave'. In Tantra Yoga, the union of yoga is therefore seen as the union of the *Kundalini* energy with pure consciousness, the final objective of all yogic endeavors.

When the *Kundalini* energy is awakened and moves upwards

---

[152] '*Hridaya*', also known as the spiritual heart.

[153] The '*Bhramara Gufa*', yet consciousness is not really located in any particular place in the body or the universe, as it is omnipresent. It is attached there through the intermediary of *Nadis*.

through the *Chakra*s, the experience of consciousness is gradually withdrawn from the more gross bodies to the more subtle bodies, until it reaches the bliss of the Self. As the veils of our different bodies are withdrawn, identification with these aspects of our being is dropped, until we experience full identification with the Self.

This wonderful story has probably given rise to the most incorrect and imaginary ideas and practices that can be found within the yoga community. The rising of the *Kundalini* energy through the *Chakra*s only happens in real deep meditation or sometimes in other real states of trance[154]. Any other movements of energy that we can produce and experience are not really movements of *Kundalini*.

All kinds of visualizations and imaginations regarding the movement of *Kundalini* while still being in a normal waking state are basically incorrect. Solar, lunar and neutral energies are continuously moving through the *Chakra*s and all kinds of valuable techniques exist with which this movement can be controlled, and channels can become unblocked. *Pranic* energy can even be felt directly when holding the palm of the hand over the 7th *Chakra*[155], but that again is not *Kundalini*. Gems, colors, sounds, etc. can be used to influence all these energies moving through the *Chakra*s, but they are entirely useless when it comes to directly affecting *Kundalini*.

As we balance the desires of the *Chakra*s as explained above, this spiritual progress will bring a natural upward movement of our attention and identification, which prepares us for a real *Kundalini* experience. But for *Kundalini* to even just leave the first *Chakra*, body consciousness as the experience of sitting somewhere must be absent.

---

[154] Such states of trance are known to come in a variety of ways, such as through extreme emotions, exhaustion or the use of certain psychedelics.

[155] Hold the middle of the palm of the hand a few centimeters above the crown *chakra*.

The actual *Kundalini Yoga* is a highly specialized technique, combining breath with certain physical locks[156] that are maintained through particular body movements and postures. It produces the fusion of the negative ions of pure *Prana* with the positive ions of *Apana*. This fusion generates a tremendous energy that awakens the snake, forcing the *Kundalini* to rise. So, we might say it is a shortcut, but one still has to be ready for it. To avoid any physical and mental imbalances as a result of this technique, the body, the energy channels and the different forms of *Prana* must be properly cleaned and balanced before it can be safely used. It may nevertheless create extraordinarily strong experiences of detachment during the meditation practice, that later may enter into conflict with less matured desires. Maybe the experience will bring one a very deep understanding of the futility in seeking some kind of emotional release in sexuality, while sexual desire may still be very much present. Overall spiritual progress is still required.

The most natural and durable way to make the *Kundalini* energy rise is 'simply' through deep meditation. If our energies are more or less balanced, and we can keep mind withdrawn and in silence long enough for body consciousness to disappear, the *Kundalini* will rise. Any such experience will fundamentally alter our personality and identification, cleaning away remaining impurities and attachments. The cumulative effect of such experiences ultimately leads to the very end point of the game.

---

[156] Named '*Bhandas*'.

8
OUR SOUL

The question remains who is the one playing this yoga game of reuniting consciousness and energy, allowing to merge individual consciousness into cosmic consciousness? Who is identifying with the various manifestations of the seeds of the Self and hence desires to bring Sound, Space and Time in balance through practice ?

Seeing the Self as the only ultimate reality, it may seem that this question is not particularly relevant. And yet it is not the Self who is actually playing this game. It is always in our presence silently beckoning us to join it, yet the Self does not make a move. One might say that the Self has the easiest job in the universe, as there is nothing it needs to do but exist. The true hero of the game of yoga is our dear ego, while at the same time the ego is the primary obstruction on the yogic path.

There cannot be any real path to the Self, as we already are that Self. In that way, there can be no plan, no process, no progress, no technique, no path. And yet in learning to stay with the Self, which in truth is so amazingly easy to find, there is a path. Because that which is always drawing us away from the Self is the illusion of individuality or ego created by the play of energy. To increasingly balance the energy, resolve any blockages, and dissolve that delusion most definitely is a matter of progress. The path is not needed to reach the Self. It is there to gradually lose the ego. There is nothing to be attained or acquired, as the Self is always in our presence. Yet there is a path that leads us away from delusion, slowly but surely. Practitioners cannot be robbed of this very real opportunity to progress, which originates in the very seeds of the Self. If one discounts the turns, it is a straight path. That path is just as much part of the truth as always focusing on the Self is. It consists of a variety of practices related to the main manifestations of the seeds of the Self, bringing our energy closer to the feeling of the Self.

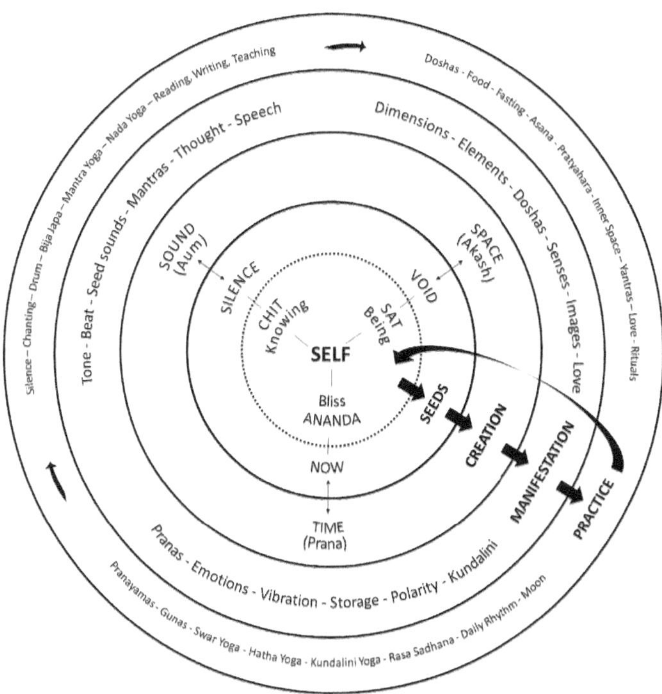

*ill. 20. - Main Manifestations of the Seeds of the Self
and the related Practices.*

The people that are so obsessed these days about the difference between a direct path and a progressive path should realize that these are not truly opposites. The opposite of a progressive path is an instant path, which is not a path at all, but rather the immediate withdrawal into the now of the Self. The direct path promoted by nonduality teachers still includes the idea of progress, otherwise it would not be named a path. Why else would Ramana Maharishi often refer to the ancient seven steps towards enlightenment[157] ? A gradual letting go of attachments is simply complementary to the ever-increasing ability to instantly return to the bliss and peace of the Self.

Wanting to jump in one master move from the intellectual understanding of the Self to the real pure enlightened beingness is not only a matter of misunderstanding or naivety. It is in itself just another ego game. We see the solution to all our troubles and we want it now. Yet, as our manifested existence contains the many different layers of our various bodies, the ego has so many different levels of identification. To peel away each layer only reveals the next one. It is a process that takes time, just like a snake will only shed its skin when it is ready. The subconscious mind is the final layer before we actually reach the body of the Self and can fully identify with it.

THE SUBCONSCIOUS

We can compare the subconscious to a cellar. Whatever stuff we find in life that we cannot effectively use, digest, recycle or discard, we throw it in our cellar. Our house seems clean, yet our cellar is still full of smelly, noisy junk. The cellar door always stands somewhat ajar, however hard we try to close it. As long as that haunted cellar is not cleared out, our house does not truly feel clean. The rubbish is just hidden from sight for a while.

---

[157] The '*Bhumikas*', see further in this chapter.

Likewise, whatever feeling comes to us that we cannot handle, we tend to suppress it. By forcing our consciousness away from it, we push it into the subconscious. Yet, that does not mean that we are free from it. The vibration of these suppressed emotions will continuously generate new feelings and thoughts in the conscious mind. Karmically speaking, that same vibration will even produce the triggers or challenges needed in life to bring them back to the conscious mind[158], where they can be properly processed and released. Especially whenever we silence the conscious mind, the subconscious will try to fill the emptiness with feelings related to past impressions[159]. Our willpower can block that from happening and when meditating, that is the right thing to do. Yet, it is no real solution, just the postponement of a process that needs to happen anyway. Any durable spiritual progress really occurs as a letting go of things within the subconscious mind, no matter how vigorously our conscious mind resists that idea.

As opposed to the conscious frontal brain, western science locates the subconscious in the midbrain and hindbrain. And sure, apart from the automation of certain bodily functions, there we also find the neural patterns that represent old, hidden memories alongside rather primitive instinctive responses that originate with our animal nature. Territorial behavior for instance, is very much fueled by the reptilian brain. Yet, the subconscious is not limited to the more remote parts of our brain. According to yogic science, it is mostly present within our very soul.

People often confuse the words soul and Self, while they are entirely different concepts. While the Self is impersonal, the soul is still

---

[158] Karma ever remains one of the greatest mysteries, about which I hope to one day write another book.

[159] The '*Vasanas*' or past impressions, desires and emotions.

very personal. The soul[160] is the subtle energy body[161] that moves from one physical body to the next in the process of reincarnation. With the body of bliss and the Self at its very center, it mostly consists of the body of the subconscious[162], but including the seed of the conscious mind.

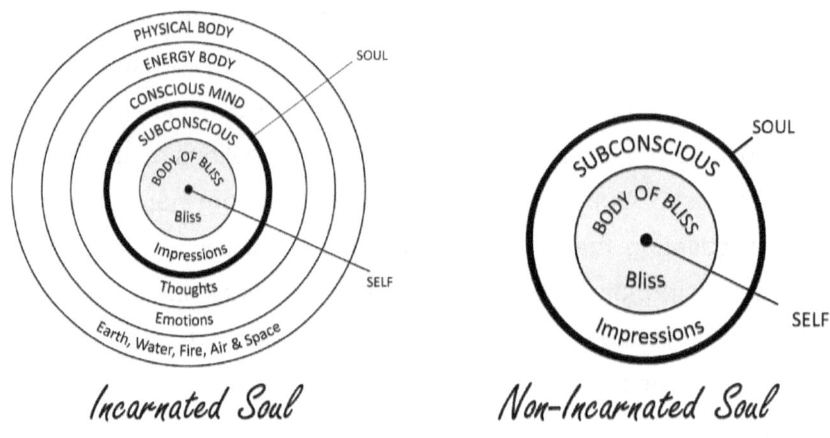

ill. 21. - Incarnated and Non-Incarnated Souls.

In the soul we find all our memories, as well as a large variety of attachments, producing deep feelings of attraction or repulsion. There we find the most original forms of the ego, in the principal ideas of being this or that aspect of our manifested beingness. Spiritual progress in terms of shedding the different layers of our ego attachments thus most essentially is a process within our subconscious soul, happening through many experiences and indeed many lives. This is directly related to the energy channels and

---

[160] The '*Jiva*', or 'being made of breath'.

[161] The energy body of the soul is said to be the size of a thumb.

[162] '*Vijnanamayi Kosha*', the 'body of knowledge'.

centers[163], that connect the body of the soul to our less subtle bodies.

Typical teachings on nonduality obviously tend to disregard the evolutions in the subconscious and the soul. Any question on past or future lives is seen as a deviation from the direct path, a distraction created by the ego. And yet, the same seers who brought us the joyful message of the Self equally describe the wonderful process of reincarnation as the way in which the soul may gradually merge with the Self. Seeing and accepting ourselves as a work in progress, as a soul on the path of gradually but surely becoming more light, can bring so much peace. We are free to take our time, as many lives as we see fit. The sense of hurry produced by the idea to have to grasp the final goal this very instant or never, then disappears. Even though full of obstacles, the path of progress is clear, a natural process of letting go.

NATURAL GROWTH

As the tree grows towards the light, our soul will slowly, slowly mature and direct its energy and awareness upward. We gradually become more transparent and let the light of the Self shine through. One beautiful way in which to comprehend this process is through the naturally maturing desires (see also illustration 22) related to the elements of our seven main energy centers or *Chakras*[164]:

1. The desire for security in the first *Chakra* always leads to stress, as security can never be 100 %, and the work seems never truly done.

2. When people then feel somewhat secure through their work,

---

[163] See Chapter 7.

[164] See also 'The Desires of the Chakras' on youtube.com/youyoga.

desire naturally evolves towards relaxation from this stress by having some fun, the second *Chakra* desire for pleasure.

3. After a while, too much partying becomes boring, and the desire manifests to achieve something, be someone important, which is the third *Chakra* desire. Through a lot of work and depending on *Karma*, we may then attain a higher social status.

4. As it is lonely at the top, we experience the emptiness of status and outward achievements, so the fourth *Chakra* desire develops to actually be loved instead of only being respected. As a result of opening our heart and deepening our connections, the sufferings of our loved ones then become our suffering as well.

5. From our compassion for others including ourselves, the fifth *Chakra* desire for more understanding is born, hoping to better protect the happiness of our loved ones. After a significant amount of study, we come to the conclusion that the actual solution is not in understanding, but in a different kind of being, a happiness that remains independent from what happens. The resulting feeling of wonder silences our thought process, and we move from thinking to non-thinking.

6. We want to achieve the true aim of yoga, which is the merging of the ego with the Self to produce ever-lasting happiness. So at some point, yoga and meditation become our main hobby, as we want nothing less than enlightenment, the desire of the sixth *Chakra*.

7. The more we progress there, the more we may detach and achieve the desireless state of the crown or seventh *Chakra*, moving beyond the elements.

The evolution of desires through the *chakras* towards essentially more satisfying levels is a natural process, which nobody can escape.

In the end, everyone is predestined to become enlightened, in this life or another. So relax, it is our freedom to let go of all these less essential desires, which in part happens by fulfilling them. Then we can really experience them as less essential and always finally resulting in some kind of unhappiness. *Tantra Yoga* holds desire as a sacred expression of the life force and sees the artful and harmonious fulfillment of desires as the natural means to move beyond. Even if we only want enlightenment, still desire will be needed to provide us with the energy to go for it.

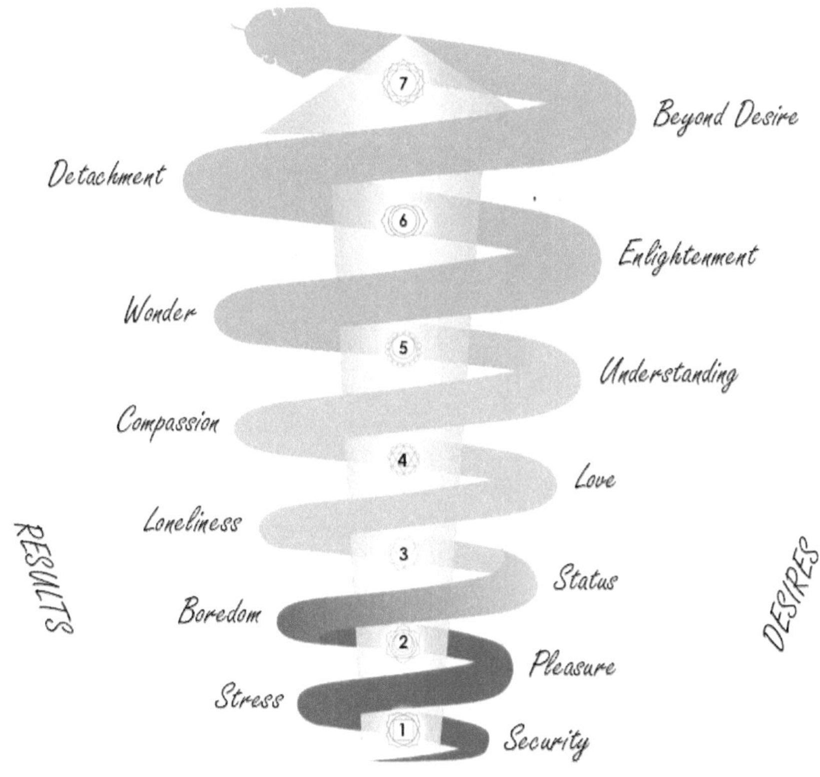

ill. 22. - Naturally Maturing Desires of the Chakras.

Yet another beautiful way to see the naturalness of spiritual progress is found in the very logical seven ancient steps or phases towards enlightenment[165], which were also very much brought forward by Sri Ramana Maharishi :

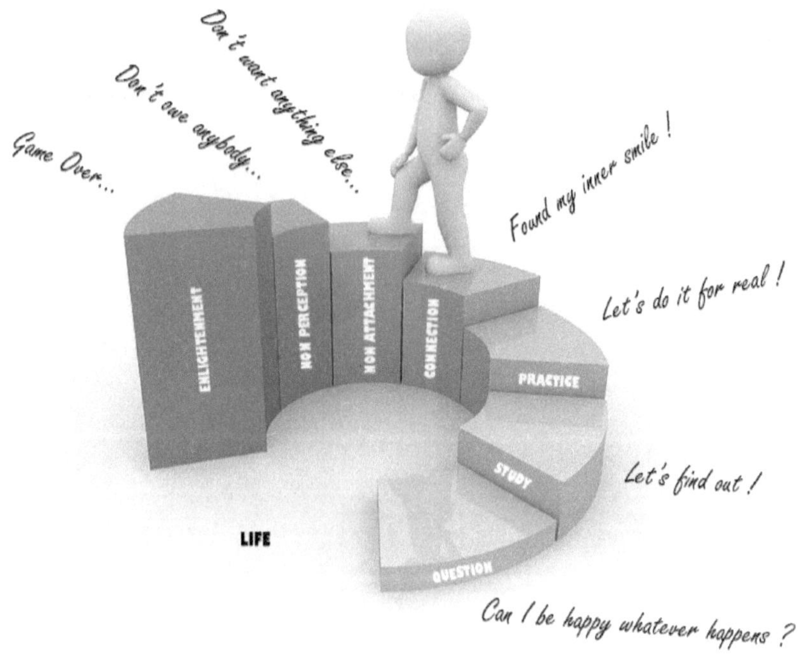

ill. 23. - Spiritual progress involves lots of dancing up and down these seven ancient steps towards enlightenment.

1. Auspicious Desire : The game of yoga starts with the desire to be happy whatever happens, the 6th *Chakra* desire.

2. Self-Inquiry : The second phase leads us to study this desire, revealing the different yogic paths and the blockages upon these

---

[165] The '*Bhumikas*', originally found in the Varaha Upanishads, see also 'Seven Steps to Enlightenment' on youtube.com/youyoga.

paths.

3. Thinning Mind : The third phase comes when we put the theory into practice and start meditating earnestly.

4. Self-Realization : In the fourth phase, we have found our inner smile through sufficient connection with the Self in deep meditation. Ramana translates this phase as Self-realization[166]. It means that we can already be happy whenever we want, because we have the ability to instantly reconnect to the endless source of happiness that is the Self and have fully mastered the *Sattvic* feeling. We may then most harmoniously fulfill our remaining desires in this phase, which may take quite a while.

5. Non-Attachment : In the fifth phase, we have fulfilled any remaining desires and become totally non-attached to anything but the Self. What remains to be done is the full payment of our still outstanding karmic debts.

6. Non-Perception : In the sixth phase, no more debts are left, and we stop perceiving the outside world, having no more interest nor duty there.

7. Liberation : After a while, this naturally leads to the seventh and last phase of enlightenment or liberation, where the sense of individuality is entirely lost, and only pure cosmic conscious energy remains.

A very important understanding here is that forceful detachment is only very much needed in phase three. There we really need to detach to have the full experience of the Self in deep meditation, so that we develop the power to be happy independent of what

---

[166] That is what it really means, while it is often confused with 'enlightenment' or '*Moksha*'.

happens[167]. Afterwards, fulfilling our desires in detached attachment[168] again becomes essential for progress in phase four, until we become really non-attached to any desires in phase five. Detachment means that we are still attached, yet we willfully push that attachment away. Non-attachment is no longer forceful, a natural state.

Another lesson to learn is that, while selfless service becomes the main practice only in the fifth phase, it always pays to spend some time on it also in the earlier phases. This way, our karmic debts will not only already be much reduced by the time we become non-attached to any personal desires. Our karmic records will then also not so much disturb the fulfillment of our own desires in phase four. Until phase five however, we are as much responsible to help ourselves, as we are to help others.

The main gem to take away from understanding these seven stages is to see how naturally joyful life already becomes in the fourth phase of Self-realization. Minor ripples on the surface of our emotional balance may still occur, but can be easily resolved whenever we want. Enlightenment may not be possible to reach in this life, due to the need to let go of an unknown number of karmic impressions and related duties. Many of those we may remain unaware off until they manifest. Yet, for sure it is possible for anyone in this very life to reach the fourth phase where we have sufficient Self-connection to become masters of our *Sattvic* feeling. Then life becomes truly an wonderful game and enlightenment can wait. All that it requires is the regular temporary detachment from everything but the Self in phase three, a few years of sincere and suitable

---

[167] '*Sattvapatti*, meaning 'ruler of *Sattva*' – see Chapter 7.

[168] See also 'Detached Attachment' on youtube.com/youyoga.

practice only, for most.

THE DARK NIGHT OF THE SOUL

While the subconscious soul is the layer of individuality that is closest to the Self, it is at the same time the layer that most strongly obscures the light of the Self. Through real deep meditation the blockages within the subconscious can be dissolved in the light of the Self, after which they can be finally fully overcome through conscious actions in life itself[169]. Deep meditation may however not yet be attainable, and some of these memories from childhood or past lives may be too painful, too obscure to be removed in this way. The subconscious is then experienced as a 'pain body', even though it also holds very beautiful memories and attachments. Recognizing this pain body may be very helpful in distancing ourselves from it, yet that may not be enough to silence it.

Some blockages are known to basically make deep meditation impossible, destroying all hard-won peace by producing sudden raw overwhelming emotions such as anger or fear while meditating. They may cause us to freeze into inaction, appearing as real obstructions that stop us from behaving in life as we would want. Such memories may need some real digging in, bringing them back to the surface of the conscious mind. There they can be properly digested in better understanding of what actually happened and why. This is often called the shadow work or entering the 'Dark Night of the Soul', which is an old Roman Catholic idea that gained new popularity these days.

There is a lot of misunderstanding on the nature of this process.

---

[169] This is the essential complementarity between the 'Path of Shiva' that leads us inside, and the 'Path of Vishnu' that brings the inside outside.

Many people are complaining about how hard awakening is, while awakening to reality is not a terrible thing, it is beautiful. When it is experienced as shameful or frightening, there is too much emphasis on the discovery of what we are not, and too little real energetic connection to that which we are. True awakening means the really hilarious discovery of our divine Self. It produces laughter without end precisely because the ego is revealed as a nonexistent drama clown, however persistent and convincing its unhappiness may be.

Realizing the many obstacles that the ego throws on the path does not need to lead us into despair, when the ego is correctly understood to be as natural as our hands and feet. Without the ego, how can we even move those hands and feet? If we would not somehow identify with being a human, we might as well try to catch salmon in an ice-cold river, with the furry paws that we don't have. Like the body, the ego is a vehicle allowing us to play the game of life. Without some ego, any action becomes impossible. To act, we need to be like actors who believe in their roles, yet preferably not forgetting our actual identity.

The ego-bashing that is so popular these days has led me to write the booklet 'Love Your Ego'[170]. It concludes as follows[171] : 'Our ego can be trouble or bliss. The only one who causes trouble about the ego is the ego itself. Condemning the ego is asking for trouble. Loving the ego is bliss. Why not simultaneously accept our imperfection as well as our eternal opportunity for growth towards perfection? If we can accept that the ego and the Self exist simultaneously within manifestation, then we are at least halfway there. Be the Self and be yourself, that's it. We do not need to be perfect. We are the art of life,

---

[170] 'Love your Ego: as you love your Self', by Peter Marchand, independently published 2019.

[171] This is a synthesized version of the last chapter.

the purpose of creation. Each second counts as an eternity, an absolutely unique step in the universal dance. The Self loves our ego as itself, sees no difference. How can we live from the Self if we cannot accept the ego as the Self does? Connect heaven and earth. Be like an arrow shot from the heart.'

Some people have called this book on our beloved ego particularly compassionate. I disagree, and this not only because self-love is key to the spiritual process. It is very clear when observing people that however dire or pleasant the circumstances, we may still choose to smile or not. Nevertheless, while the feeling of suffering or enjoyment is thus an illusion, it does not feel that way. For that reason, one cannot be compassionate enough in accepting that our dear little ego child needs some help on the way towards accepting its divine nature. It not only requires the light of truth to show the way, but also the power of love and compassion motivating it to move forward.

FEEDING THE LIGHT

Having discovered the beauty of the Self, we truly owe it to ourselves to be reconciled with our dear ego. If then we feel the need to enter deep into the darkest corners of our soul, we should bring our light along[172]. The despair of the Catholic seekers on discovering their ultimate smallness, causing shame and a desire for redemption, originates with the idea of a perfect divinity existing only outside of them. Let us not make that same mistake. We are the Self and as individual egos we are just little children born from the Self, growing from the Self, towards the Self, into the Self. We need to let our light of love, forgiveness and truth shine in those dark corners and in order

---

[172] See also 'The Dark Night of the Soul' on youtube.com/youyoga.

to do that, first we need to make it strong.

Faced with the light of the Self, these seemingly powerful attachments only have the power that we attribute to them or not. Some 'Dark Night of the Soul' session may be useful or even needed but should first include whatever practice we have developed to generate our unlimited divine power. Otherwise, it will only strengthen those attachments, deepen the darkness. From the sweetness that we find within our deepest being, it becomes very easy to forgive, easy to forget, natural to let go.

Very basic here is the wisdom that in the game of life, pleasure cannot exist without the presence of pain. The tongue that enjoys the taste of chocolate is the tongue that does not like the taste of shit. If everything would be white, nothing could be seen. And while we might hope for everyone to be 'good', nobody can be good without the freedom to be bad. Honesty can only be if dishonesty is an option. No Buddha is possible without the potential of a Hitler. No life without death. No pain, no pleasure. As the kid who gets hurt in soccer yet still wants to play, we can accept the pain in return for the pleasure. Whatever pain we find within the darkest corners of our soul, we can accept it to be there and then accept that it does not need to stay, letting it go, disidentifying.

Identification with our divine light is the key to let it shine within all layers of our soul. In as far as our essential identity is understood but not felt, we need to transform the very energy of this soul body. While the tree cannot be found within the seed, it is from the tree that we can produce the seeds we need. We use the powers of Sound, Space and Time until there will be no more darkness obscuring the light. Using the power of mantra, breath or the inner senses are examples of how our soul can be healed on the energetic level, which is needed for any acceptance to become real.

BIRTH & REBIRTH

For the one who does not believe in reincarnation[173], discovering the complexity of our ego attachments truly can feel like a one-way trip to hell. How can we ever trust in our ability to weed out all of that in just one lifetime? The much-praised idea of 'only living once' actually brings a lot of stress to people. We tend to always doubt that reincarnation story somehow, because we usually have no direct experience of it. A quite natural power of ignorance or delusion[174] keeps us from seeing the truth of our rebirth. Through a variety of practical experiences, we may finally accept it. One might moreover study the many reports about people who do have some memory of their past lives and have ways to prove it.

Sometimes unhappiness leads to the idea of needing to escape from this cycle of death and rebirth, which became like a religion to many people. The true path of yoga is to escape from the illusion of unhappiness and separation, powered by embracing the cycle of death and rebirth, which is at our very disposal to succeed. Of course, the ego may love the idea of many lives. That does not however make it untrue.

To experience ourselves as souls with eternity at our disposal for growth, brings such relief. No more hurry or worry, no need for shame or guilt, plenty of room for making errors, enough time to explore and cleanse that dark maze of the subconscious. Timelessness also to

---

[173] By far, my greatest personal benefit from interacting with the spiritual world through the art of healing has been the deep realization and acceptance of the truth of reincarnation. It brought the blissful assurance of having all the time that I need to work on myself.

[174] This veiling power of *Maya* or illusion is natural and needed, otherwise how could a tiger behave naturally if in its last life it was a deer?

fulfill any remaining natural desires in life[175], wasting eternal time the good way. Every new life is a chance to let go of the last. With every new body comes a new identity. When our suit feels patched beyond repair, we can get a new one for free. Such wealth, such blessing, such happy gratitude.

Accepting the reality of reincarnation brings up questions about some of the more specific purposes of this particular life that we find ourselves living. How does it relate to our past lives and what do we want to achieve in this one? The subconscious affected the choices we made for this life, while being in between lives. As souls do not have a brain, these choices are not made very rationally. They are more of an emotional, vibrational nature, karmic powers that pull us this way or the other.

Various levels of our being are involved, that create certain powers that attract us to a particular fetus, a family, a country. Love is the queen of these powers, bringing us back to some other beings to whom we feel connected, or to some skill or talent that we would like to develop further. Child prodigies are examples of souls who have brought with them highly developed talents and are usually entirely focused on further exploring them throughout their lives. Most people have more diverse desires when they reincarnate, and their path may thus not be so clear or focused. While some divinatory sciences may shed more light on this question[176], our emotional triggers are key indicators, as they point to deeper attachments that seem not to have been born during this life. In entirely disregarding the ego, we may purposefully ignore the very reasons why we were in fact born again. Accepting these karmic attachments and fulfilling those very deep

---

[175] My childhood dream of once reaching the very top of Mount Everest will most probably not be fulfilled in this life. I couldn't care less. One day it will happen, whether in pants or a dress.

[176] I personally mostly use numerology for that purpose in my healing and coaching practice.

desires may be a much easier way to find and keep the peace of the Self.

Even though by nature it is ever changing, our individual soul is truly eternal within manifestation. Through endless cycles of death and rebirth, we actually never die, and life just continues. And if one day we escape manifestation through enlightenment, that will be just the end page of a highly entertaining book. And it does not need to be the end. While most people tend to believe that enlightenment means that we fully disappear into cosmic beingness, that is just one option.

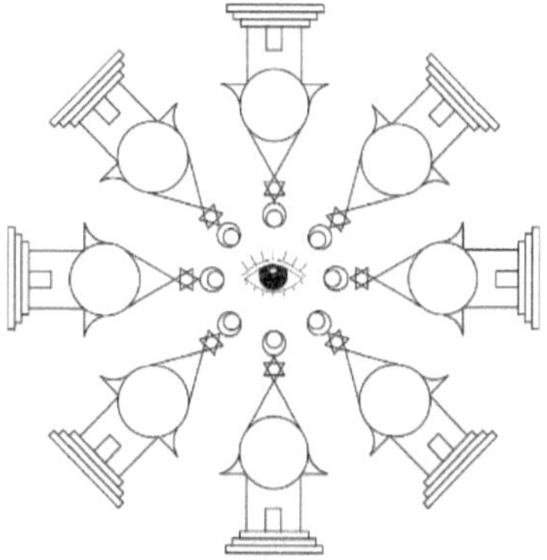

ill. 24. - All our Temples of the Body (see Chapter 6) are Connected in Nondual Cosmic Beingness through the Element of Space.

Enlightenment means absolute liberation, so the freedom for our soul to again play at life is included. Vedic scripture has numerous accounts of how various people became enlightened, only to dive right back into the game[177]. Anyhow, no hurry, as we are all together already connected through the element of Space to the nondual cosmic beingness. We just tend to forget it.

---

[177] See for example, 'The Supreme Yoga: A New Translation of the Yoga Vāsiṣṭha', by Venkates Ananda Saraswati, Motilal Banarsidass 2001.

9
SPIRITUAL DIMENSIONS

Acceptance of the truth of reincarnation brings with it the logical question of where and how the journey of the soul from one physical body to the next is happening? Many people who like to believe in reincarnation have trouble in accepting the idea of spirits or a spiritual world. And yet, without spirits existing in a spiritual world, reincarnation could not happen. The belief in a spiritual reality beyond the material world is what truly separates 'spiritual people' from others.

Vedic cosmology then points to the presence of other dimensions[178] beyond the physical world. Just as the Earth element contains water and all other elements without those being immediately apparent, the Earth dimension hides other dimensions that are contained within. This phenomenon can be compared to a Russian doll hiding other Russian dolls inside, each again hiding the next.

The truth is that while we have the impression of being here in the physical dimension, our souls actually exist within another dimension. Taking on a physical body does not mean to become that body or even to move inside of it. It means that from a more subtle dimension that is hidden within the physical dimension, the soul connects to the

---

[178] The '*Lokas*', planes of existence.

physical body through energetic channels or cords[179], connected with the *Chakras*. They produce the experience of being here and allow us to use the physical body. We are 'simply' playing a perfect kind of virtual reality game within a complex energetic matrix. Just like virtual reality helmets do, these energetic 'wires' remove the experience of actually existing in some other spiritual dimension, even though that is where our soul really resides. We are free to choose the blue pill over the red one[180].

Leaving the physical body upon death then simply means to withdraw our life force from those energetic cords, again revealing our existence as souls within another dimension. Before reincarnating by making a connection to a new physical body, that then also allows our souls to first travel to yet other spiritual dimensions. There we can have different kinds of experiences that may be highly beneficial to our spiritual growth.

The truth of the soul and the spiritual worlds is often regarded as an inconveniently obscure truth. Here we need to rely on faith to motivate us to engage in at least some practical experience, through which that faith may become a real knowing. As long as the direct experience in deeper meditation lies beyond our grasp, we can try out – in the correct and heartfelt way - some more basic ritual practice and await the result. Then we may come to accept that spiritual world to exist, even while remaining beyond our understanding.

There are so many things in the physical world that we accept to exist, even though we do not fully understand them, like how a seed grows into a tree. Science may describe how many things work in nature, but this understanding has yet to bring us a scientist that can

---

[179] '*Nadis*' or energy channels, which are found both within the physical body as outside of it.

[180] Referring to the movie 'The Matrix', where this basic idea is quite well represented, even if instead of a soul, the physical body is connected to the illusion of life in that story.

actually create a seed from which a tree will grow. From a different perspective, the physical dimension may be seen as even more magical, more difficult to understand than the more subtle dimensions. Our senses actually make the physical dimension appear as real and the spiritual dimensions as unreal. As we now primarily live within the physical dimension, that also makes a lot of sense. Yet sometimes it may be wise to look beyond the senses and accept that also other realities are at play.

VEDIC COSMOLOGY

The spiritual dimensions[181] are directly related to the elements hidden within the Earth element that constitutes the physical dimension[182]. As such they are very special expressions of the mother matter of Space, that emerged from the seed of *Sat* in the Self. Water, Fire, Air and Space are relatively formless, as only the Earth element has the density needed to create any fixed forms. It is from these formless elements that the body of our soul is made. Like a cloud, the energy body of the soul can thus take on different shapes. And like a cloud also, the energy body of the soul can become more subtle and light, which allows it to travel to more subtle dimensions related to the more subtle elements.

The first dimension where a soul finds itself after 'leaving' the physical body is the astral world[183], connected to the water element. It is closely related to the Plane of Fantasy[184], as everything that we

---

[181] See much more detail in 'The Yoga of Snakes and Arrows: The Leela of Self-Knowledge' by Harish Johari, Destiny Books 2007.

[182] '*Bhu Loka*', the 'physical plane'.

[183] '*Bhuvar Loka*', the 'astral plane'.

[184] '*Naga Loka*', the 'plane of Fantasy', which also relates to snakes as symbols of desire.

can imagine in this dimension appears as real. Equally in dreaming, that is where we have our experiences. Like a country may have many regions, each dimension has many different 'places' to explore, which are not dimensions in themselves[185]. Some souls may prefer to stay in the astral dimension for a long time or even travel to other dimensions. Such 'traveling' however again must be seen as a further withdrawal to the center of our being, to our ever more subtle energy bodies. Many souls will however rather rapidly reincarnate from the astral world, reconnecting to the physical world.

Within the astral world there is the next even more subtle dimension of the celestial world[186], which is related to the fire element and is called the first heaven. It is said to house luminous beings made of fire or light, which depending upon culture may be called angels, deities[187] or saints. Also more 'common' souls may visit this dimension, in as far as they are able to detach from the less subtle dimensions, which is a matter of desire.

It really goes beyond the scope of this book to fully describe all the other truly mysterious dimensions beyond that first heaven[188]. They each hold different 'regions' and are ever more subtle until they no longer relate to one of the five elements. Then they are even said to escape the creation and destruction of different universes, which only happens on the level of the elements[189]. Illustration 25 shows how the Physical Plane can be seen as holding all other dimensions within

---

[185] Even though they are also named '*Lokas*', such as '*Pitr Loka*', '*Yaksha Loka*', or '*Rasa Loka*'.

[186] '*Swarga Loka*', the 'celestial plane'.

[187] We usually translate the Sanskrit '*Devata*' as deities or gods and goddesses, yet it is actually a much broader term for spiritual energies.

[188] Named '*Maha Loka*', '*Jana Loka*', '*Tapah Loka*' and '*Satya Loka*'.

[189] The dimensions that are said to escape the destruction of the 'elemental' universe are '*Tapah Loka*' and '*Satya Loka*', and of course also the dimension of the Absolute.

itself or having all other dimensions stacked 'on top' of it. This image is not meant to express reality, only to show how our experience may change according to our point of view, seeing either a narrowing tunnel or a cone. All indeed depends on how our eyes change perspective, placing the Self either on top of all other dimensions, or at the very center of them.

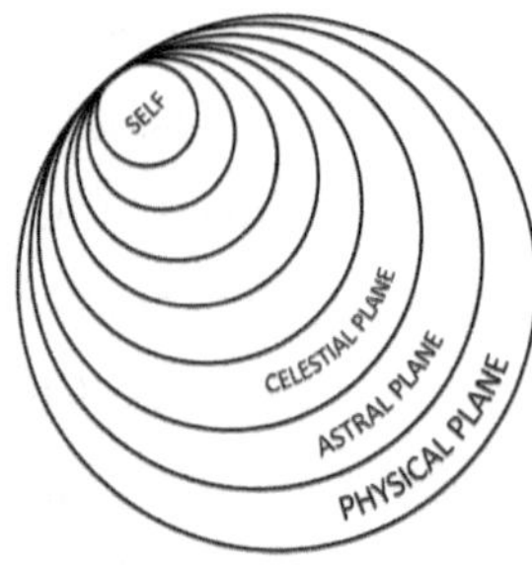

ill. 25. Perspective and the Experience of the Spiritual Dimensions.

Worth mentioning of course is the Absolute Dimension[190] of the Self. This is a place that is no place, as it is said to be equally present within all dimensions. It is absolute, beyond any duality of here or there. This nondual dimension pervades and encompasses all other manifested dimensions and truly makes them one, overruling any importance given to any other dimension.

SPIRITUAL TRAVELS & EXPERIENCES

Whether incarnated or not, we thus exist simultaneously within different, ever more subtle dimensions. As such, our soul can be

---

[190] Depending on the chosen form of the divine, this dimension is named '*Vaikunta Loka*', '*Brahma Loka*', *Rudra Loka*' or even '*Prakriti Loka*'.

described as a fine, intricate, multidimensional galaxy of energy channels and centers, which connect to the elements and to the sheaths of consciousness[191]. It may be hard to imagine ourselves that way, yet this description comes quite close to describing what we really are as individuals.

In deep meditation, we first withdraw from the physical dimension, when the experience of sitting somewhere in a physical body fully disappears. We then enter the imaginary astral world, which may lead to certain more or less distracting audiovisual experiences. As our meditation deepens, we may withdraw from the concrete inner mental objects of our meditation such as *mantras* or *yantras*. We then move towards more abstract and subtle energetic objects existing in the even more subtle dimensions[192].

This is the actual meaning of the rising of the *Kundalini* energy through the *Chakras*. When the *Kundalini* leaves the Earth element of the first *Chakra*, we withdraw our energy and awareness from the physical dimension into the astral world. When we, as *Kundalini*, move beyond the water element of the second *Chakra*, we have withdrawn to our more luminous form within the celestial world, etc.

This explains the many reports of people going to unusual places and meeting different beings in deep meditation. If indeed all experience of the physical world is lost, and we are not simply entertaining some mental fantasy, those meditation experiences are not illusions. Deep meditation means to gradually lift the veils that hide the other realities or dimensions within ourselves and the universe.

Even though most people are unaware of it, the spiritual

---

[191] See Chapter 2.

[192] The concrete objects such as mantras or yantras are reduced to their rather formless but distinct energetic essences.

dimensions do not only exist. They also interact quite significantly with our lives here in the physical world, precisely because on a more subtle level we do exist in those other dimensions. And this interaction can be either a blessing or a curse, which has led to the development of many practices to optimize our relationships within these spiritual worlds. As spiritual growth happens most essentially on the subconscious level of our soul, these relationships can make the difference between lengthy stagnation or rapid evolution.

A variety of spiritual connections exist through different energetic cords, which can be a source of agreeable or disagreeable feelings, seemingly triggered from the subconscious without obvious reason. What we experience as originating within the subconscious does not only come from 'our' subconscious. Through the energetic cords that connect us to the spiritual world, we are part of a 'common mind-field', which affects us much more intensely than we can imagine. It is just another way in which we are truly One.

'Like attracts like' is the main rule that governs our spiritual energy connections. A talented musician may thus gain a real spiritual audience, which may also inspire that musician as so-called 'muses'. When in meditation we successfully produce a genuinely nice *Sattvic* feeling, other spiritual beings with similar taste may enjoy it and even join in, so that an even deeper bliss can be experienced. Unfortunately this rule also applies to unpleasant emotions. If for some time a person is angry, then that may naturally attract other more angry spiritual beings. If then that person wants to let go of the anger, it may be more difficult as the energy of those spiritual beings may continue to fuel angry thoughts[193].

---

[193] In spiritual healing, removing the connection with those spiritual beings is the first thing to do in order to heal persistent unpleasant emotions.

In this way, our spiritual life is not very different from socializing in the physical world. And as in the 'real' world there are more and less agreeable people, equally in the spiritual world it is not all 'love and light'. Some really unhappy spiritual beings can be very naughty, trying to dominate us by affecting our body and mind in rather unpleasant ways, exploiting the energetic gates of the *Chakras*.

Even the people with whom we live in the physical world are connected to us through similar energetic cords, especially if strong emotional bonds exist. They may thus subconsciously influence our emotions, even if they are not physically nearby. Other more personal relationships exist in the spiritual world with the ancestor spirits, as well as with other departed souls that we know from this life or past lives. If upon meeting someone new, we immediately feel as if we already know them, that may very well be true.

Devotional practices to particular forms of the divine may attract spiritual beings with similar preferences[194], which may support our practice. The more advanced spiritual aspirants may benefit from insights and guidance received from achieved yogic masters, that reside in the most subtle dimensions. Last but not least, we have special relationships to particular karmic energies. Their function is to assure our personal contribution in maintaining balance in the universe, as well as to bring forward particular karmic impressions that produce blockages in our energy channels. In the vedic tradition, these are related to the planetary energies.

We live in a magical world, and the problem is that we usually do not perceive this magic, even if we are subject to its results. Compared to the truth of the Self, which anyone can easily experience to some degree, the magical world of our soul and its spiritual

---

[194] Through the use of particular *mantras*, *yantras* and *Pujas* or rituals.

dimensions lies beyond normal perception. Some people are born with the talent, acquired in past lives, to experience the spiritual world in the normal waking state. Some may develop it in this life if they can sufficiently detach from the physical world to explore the other dimensions in the deeper trance states.

THE PATH OF RITUAL

Just as we may be advised to breathe differently to bring our energy closer to the bliss of the Self, sometimes specific spiritual practices related to beings in the other dimensions may be extremely useful on the path of unraveling our individuality. They may consist of some more shamanic healing practices related to solving certain spiritual public relation problems with beings of a less blissful nature. Or they may be more of a devotional tantric nature, aiming to receive help from more spiritually advanced beings that support 'upward'

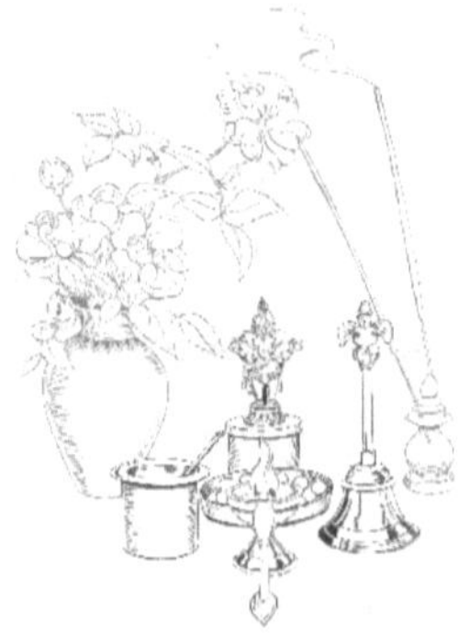

ill. 26. – Rituals are a spiritual language. (Drawing by Pieter Weltevrede)

spiritual disciplines[195], deeper meditation and the development of real intuition.

Many yogic and tantric traditions have thus developed relatively strange rituals, repeating age-old sounds and songs, creating ancient visual patterns, making certain movements according to custom and using specific offerings. All of that is truly an ancient spiritual language to communicate with spiritual beings that belonged to the same

---

[195] '*Sadhana*' meaning 'dedication to an aim'.

tradition or lineage. This explains why in different traditions rituals come in such high variety, just as languages and customs are also very different in different parts of the world. Yet, some ritual practices are more universally common throughout different traditions and cultures[196].

Many spiritual people believe that to ask for help from the spiritual world is not needed, as they expect that any more highly evolved beings will gladly provide this help whenever needed, from the kindness of their hearts. That is however not at all the case, as this would go against our essential freedom. It is our choice to meditate or not, to let go of something or hold on to it, to be angry or to be forgiving. To affect such choices would mean to rob us of our freedom of choice, and that is something that only naughty spiritual beings may try to do.

Those who can really help us on our spiritual journey will be happy to do so, if we only truly ask for it, while making our own choices. Living up to these choices may also affect it. Who can help us to see the Self if we keep looking in the other direction? We definitely do not need any such help to find the Self or stay with it. Yet, such help can be highly decisive within the process of our spiritual growth[197]. There is real support available 'up there', for the one who can bow down the ego and sincerely invite it. To expect anything particular is obviously not advisable, as karma is still involved. Expect to be guided upwards.

If we want to have some practical experience, but do not have the taste for some strange ritual that belongs to another culture,

---

[196] Such as the use of 108 prayer beads in a rosary or '*Mala*', found in Hinduism, Buddhism, Islam, Christianity, etc.

[197] It has helped me tremendously in letting go of things, as it brought deeper insights that would have been difficult to get on my own and produced overwhelming and highly motivating feelings of peace and bliss.

developing an ancestor ritual is a good place to start from. While ancestor rituals are found in all ancient cultures, they have largely disappeared in modern society. As most of my colleagues will confirm, the experience as a healer is that this basic negligence of the ancestors causes many psychological imbalances and blockages. Ancestor rituals actually come at the beginning of learning any ritual practice and since they have largely disappeared from modern culture, we are quite free to redevelop them ourselves, in the ways that we find suitable. If such rituals however still exist within our culture, then it will be most efficient to perform them just like our grandparents did.

Ancestor rituals can be really simple, as long as love for the ancestors is available, which is the chief ingredient. Basically we say, 'Hi dear ancestors, how are you doing, here are some gifts for you, please help me to be happy, healthy and wise.'. We might visualize and remember the ancestors that we have known ourselves and could ask for more specific help[198], especially for example in solving some family matters. In case we feel dislike for some ancestor, the ritual offers an ideal opportunity to see any soul as a work in progress and send that ancestor the most heartfelt good wishes.

Such ritual can take less than 5 minutes, yet it may bring quite strong improvements in one's mood, relationships and overall 'luck'. This is especially valid in families where ancestor practices have been largely absent. Even if an ancestor has already reincarnated on Earth, still their soul remains in the spiritual world just like ours does. Also for these then, an ancestor ritual may bring us some support, while their conscious mind may not be aware of giving it, being caught in the

---

[198] If we like to ask something specific, best be very clear on what we want and do not want, so there can be no wrong interpretation.

virtual reality of the physical dimension.

In a more tantric way that actually applies to most rituals, we can assure that this communication is fruitful by applying a number of simple principles that are based on the tantric science of proper communication with the spiritual world[199]:

- Rituals require regularity and optimal timing, in this case meaning that on average doing an ancestor ritual could happen for example every new moon and best in the early morning[200].

- Our mind should be clear, our stomach empty and our body clean.

- We offer some fruits, leaves and/or flowers for the Earth element, essentially providing the ancestors with the blueprints of these things. They can use them to imagine having these things in their own world, which lies just beyond the Earth element.

- We offer some fresh tap water[201] for the Water element, because water is a good energy conductor, allowing the ancestors to actually 'stay' at the place where we are performing the ritual. Offering water in a metal pot such as copper or silver works best, because metal is also highly conductive.

- We offer some fire in the form of an oil lamp or candle, because the Fire element provides the main energy to create the energetic cord needed for the ancestors to find the place where the ritual is happening, like a beacon.

- We offer some incense or essential oil for the Air element, affecting quite directly the spiritual dimension where the ancestors actually reside, strongly improving their mood.

---

[199] See my channel youtube.com/youyoga for a detailed description of ancestor rituals.

[200] See also Chapter 12. The optimal timing for other kinds of rituals may be different.

[201] Bottled water that has been standing still for a long time is not suitable, as it no longer holds the energy of 'living' water. Water from a nearby spring or river has the best quality.

- We produce some sounds in chanting or the use of bells, drums, etc. to offer the Space element, which may increase the harmony and confidence of the ancestors quite considerably.

- Having offered the 5 elements, we have in essence offered the entire universe. Any other gifts can be given, depending on cultural and personal preferences, such as some tea, tobacco or alcohol. Such more *Rajasic* or *Tamasic* gifts are not suitable for higher spiritual beings, but the more normal souls of our ancestors may very much appreciate them.

- Once these gifts are attentively arranged one by one on a plate, we can put it in nature or keep it somewhere safe inside the house. After around 24 hours, it must be returned to nature and never thrown in the dustbin.

All of this may feel quite strange at first, sure. Some doubt is very natural, yet it also means that we feel that there is a chance that we might actually help our ancestors and ourselves this way. Then why not try? If one never tries, one can never have the experience. Similar small rituals can also be performed to receive some spiritual help in meditation – see Chapter 13.

10
INTEGRAL YOGA

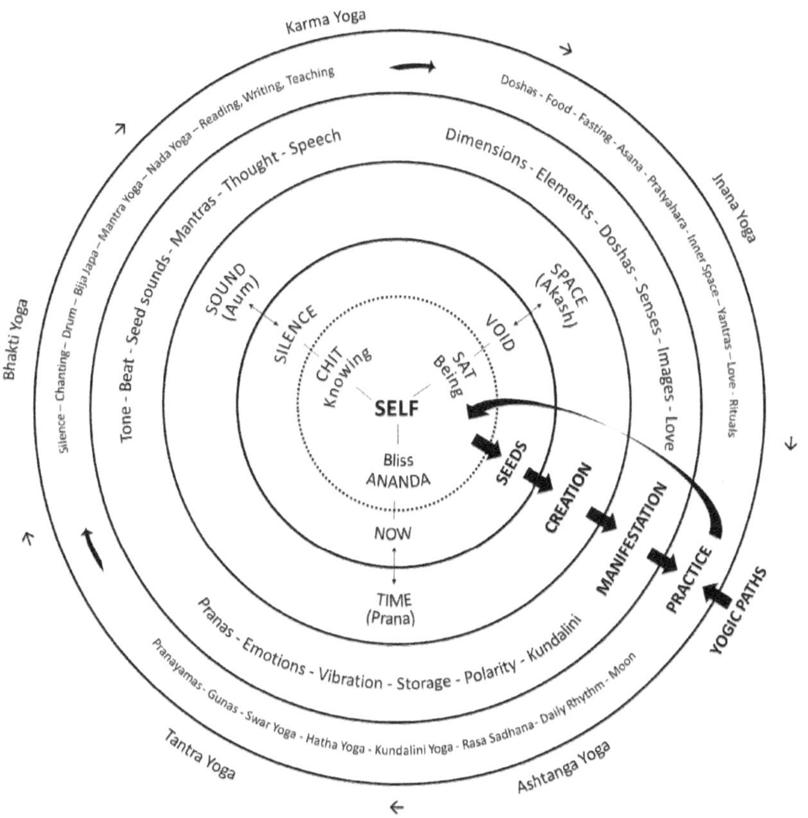

ill. 27. - The main Yogic Paths & Practices.

To generate more nondual energy in ourselves, the yogic tradition has brought us so many beautiful practices based on the seed powers of Sound, Space and Time. We definitely do not need all of them and are generally advised to develop them mostly as the need is felt. Illustration 27 gives some idea of our too many options in practice. As it pertains to our particular personality, we first choose a specific path for the ego, or a combination of the main paths. The more practical choices are usually made through such general choice of a main yogic path, in which some practices fit better than others.

PATHS FOR THE EGO

Traditionally the question on how to work with the ego is approached through the insight that people can only think, feel or act. That also brings the more yogic options of not thinking, feeling nor acting or even of doing all of that simultaneously. For each of these things that we can do, a particular essential path has been put forward by the yogic traditions.

Since we cannot truly live our daily lives without either thinking, feeling or acting, every one of us can be helped by a somewhat personal combination of these paths. In fact, one of the factors that influence this particular choice of ego-techniques is our body type, which makes us predominantly into thinkers, feelers or doers[202]. Bile dominated people are more into doing, mucus dominated people tend towards feeling, and wind dominated people like to think a lot.

So, whenever we think, we can think truth or stop thinking, which is the path of *Jnana Yoga* that focuses entirely on destroying the delusions existing in the conscious mind. Whenever we feel, we can feel unconditional love in union, which is the path of *Bhakti Yoga* or

---

[202] The '*Dosha*' or personal constitution of the physical body, see Chapter 6.

the yoga of love and devotion. Whenever we act, we can act in selfless service as opposed to any more self serving action, which is *Karma Yoga*. And whenever we want to do none of these, we apply the techniques generally known as *Ashtanga Yoga*, eight logical steps ultimately leading us into deep meditation and the end of feeling, thinking or acting. *Tantra Yoga* then - as the last of the major yogic paths - combines truth, love, selfless service and doing nothing magically into one holistic practice. Of course, we can find a multitude of different yogic traditions, each originating from particular teachers and also different parts of the world, yet these traditions all make some unique *masala* of the five main yogic paths.

These five main paths are primarily to be understood as exercises for the ego. In *Jnana Yoga*, the ego is reasoned away by questioning whatever 'I am this' it is trying to hold onto, until it identifies with the pure beingness of 'I am'. In *Bhakti Yoga*, the ego forgets itself through the feeling of love for the divine cosmic Self, that exists inside of us and everywhere else. In *Karma Yoga* the ego identifies with the needs of the entire universe in selfless service, letting go of egoic desires in the process. In *Ashtanga Yoga*, through the silencing of mind, the ego temporarily disappears, as it is essentially just the idea of separation in our thoughts. That allows for the full experience of the Self in deep meditation. In *Tantra Yoga*, all of that is being done, with the added value of unraveling particular blockages in the subconscious ego, through rather mysterious practices that work more directly with the *Kundalini* energy and improve relationships in the spiritual dimensions.

While personal preferences are logical, the true path is integral, holistic in nature. In dealing with our complex ego, we may need to take our entire manifested beingness and thus all the main paths into account. Meanwhile, reducing the ego will of course also affect our mind, energy and feelings. If the ego lets go of itself to some degree, the physical body relaxes, the *Pranic* body become lighter, the thoughts lose their edges, and even the subconscious becomes more quiet. All five yogic paths are known to stimulate feelings of love, joy, wonder, confidence and peace, while reducing anger, fear, depression and sadness.

Typical *Bhakti Yoga* practices such as chanting or rituals especially affect our energy through the loving use of sound, flowers, colors and other sensory impressions that generate positive feeling. As *Bhakti Yoga* primarily relates to feeling, it often becomes more tantric in nature, meaning that it will bring some support from the spiritual world. That is even true if our love is offered to a quite formless representation of the Self, such as the light of an oil lamp.

In a more religious context, such rituals have become ancient habits, while often the spiritual science behind them remains hidden from the participants. From the point of view of generating love, that is not unwise. Rational understanding is deadly to any finer feeling of love. While lovers may feel their love enhanced by a more romantic environment, they prefer to see their love as independent of it, truly unconditional. In the case of *Bhakti*, that is obviously also the truth, as love for the divine exists unconditionally at some level within every being. The divine is perfect, so what is there not to love?

THE EIGHT LIMBS

Any path always somehow includes some meditative practices that move us away from thinking, feeling and doing, to the non-thinking, non-feeling, non-doing pure beingness of the Self. Meditation is the ultimate way to reduce the ego's feeling of individual importance. While the methods to approach this may vary greatly, the basic meditation process has been most clearly described in the *Yoga Sutras* of Patanjali as resting upon eight sets of practices, which became known as *Ashtanga Yoga*[203]:

1. Avoiding that which removes peace[204]:

   → *Nonviolence, truth, honesty, sexual restraint, forbearance, fortitude, kindness, straightforwardness, moderation in diet, bodily purity.*

2. Focusing on that which produces peace[205]:

   → *Austerity, contentment, belief, charity, worship, study, modesty, having a discerning mind, mantra repetition, observance of vows and performing sacrifices.*

3. Sitting comfortably[206].

   → *As a motionless body makes the mind quiet, at least one sitting posture must be mastered if one is to reach and maintain a deep state of meditation.*

4. Harmonizing the pranic energy[207]:

   → *A variety of techniques including breath retention, alternate nostril breathing, Prana visualization, etc. that bring our emotional energy closer to the peace of the Self.*

5. Withdrawing inside[208]:

   → *Purification of the senses, followed by forcing our attention and the life force towards the inner senses.*

6. Inner concentration[209]:

---

[203] Literally meaning 'eight limbs', also known as the royal or '*Raja Yoga*'.

[204] '*Yama*', meaning 'to stop' or 'to kill'.

[205] '*Niyama*', meaning 'to start' or 'to make alive'.

[206] '*Asana*', meaning 'that on/in which we sit'.

[207] '*Pranayama*', meaning both 'to stop' or 'to expand' 'the life force'.

[208] '*Pratyahara*', meaning 'withdrawal from what comes in'.

[209] '*Dharana*', meaning 'concentration'.

> → *Being entirely one-pointed, focused on only one inner object.*

7. Effortless meditation[210]:

> → *Where both the object of the meditation and the power of concentration have become subtle, effortless, doerless.*

8. Absorption in deep meditation[211]:

> → *Where consciousness of the physical body disappears and nondual oneness is achieved, a mystic state of trance with many layers.*

Whatever importance the individual practitioner or particular spiritual tradition gives to each limb may differ significantly. And yet, some aspect of each limb will usually be included. *Ashtanga Yoga* is truly a holistic, integrated set of techniques that lead us to the full experience of the Self, by removing all other experiences. More on the process of meditation in Chapter 13.

TANTRIC MAGIC

Last but not least, *Tantra Yoga* can be regarded as the most integral yoga tradition, even if *Bhakti, Jnana, Karma* and *Ashtanga Yoga* can all lead to the ultimate goal on their own[212]. *Tantra Yoga* however includes all of them. Feeling love, seeing truth, selfless service and non-doing are simultaneously combined in one magical practice through the understanding of *Tantric Advaita.* What this really means is hard to explain. It can only be experienced. Definitely it

---

[210] '*Dhyana*', meaning 'to see'.

[211] '*Samadhi*', meaning 'all is perceived as one'.

[212] If pursued vigorously and smartly, that is an absolute yes.

signifies that the powers of Space, Sound and Time are put to conscious use in support of retaining Self-awareness, which is the path of the *Tantric Jnani*[213]. Tantra also facilitates the meditative journey of our soul through the spiritual dimensions, the rising of *Kundalini* and the related interactions with the spiritual world. Tantra is magical only when it thus works with the intangible, with that which is beyond understanding.

Even though I might call myself a tantric practitioner, I just as easily identify with the other paths. I would never promote *Tantra Yoga* as a yoga that serves all, especially not when it comes to the more magical practices of connecting to the spiritual world or the rising of *Kundalini.* Yet, when certain blockages are experienced in life or meditation, that seem difficult to remove with the more tangible means, we may need to work with the more intangible energies instead. Then the more mystical, occult practices of *Tantra Yoga* may become highly advisable, but these are usually quite demanding. An alternative may be found in tantric healing, where the healer offers help through the powers gained in his or her own practice. Nevertheless, the use of particular *mantras* and relatively simple cleansing rituals by the 'patients' themselves may be of great aid in the healing process.

While the objective of this book is to bring more insight into the tantric philosophy of nonduality, it was never the intent to describe the actual tantric practices here in any detail. The readers that had hoped to find those descriptions here, should accept that those are hardly suited to be taught through a book. They require a more personal relationship between student and teacher. The transfer of information is quite irrelevant in Tantra because the mysteries are in any case

---

[213] The *Tantric Jnani* is combining the unrelenting awareness of nondual consciousness with the mastery of nondual energy.

beyond understanding. Only practical experience counts, and here the teacher's role is mostly that of a guide and protector, rather than the one who spoils everything through speech in advance. The value of words here lies more in their feeling and power than in their meaning. Maybe one day I might write a book on the subject, but it truly must be rather limited. Meanwhile, whoever is truly drawn to the tantric practices may contact me in person for support.

Within this book on *Tantric Advaita*, I mostly hope to bring understanding on where and how certain more or less tantric practices might fit in. True knowing is to see the togetherness of things, which also applies to practices. For the rest I prefer to limit practical advice here to the more day-to-day uses of the powers of Sound, Space and Time. For the one who can thus balance some very basic things like breath, food, tuning into natural cycles, daily meditation, emotions, etc., awareness of Self will come much more effortlessly and that is the main objective of *Tantric Jnana*[214]. Honestly, only then the more advanced Tantric practices become attainable.

PITFALLS OF THE PATHS

For the *Jnani* or the *Tantric*, the *Bhakta*, *Ashtanga* or *Karma* yogi, the essential truth of the Self always remains the same. It is the truth of the absolute reality, the pure beingness, the oneness, the union. Only the methods in how to find, realize, maintain or live that truth are different. Unfortunately, throughout history all paths have created some tricky interpretations of the one truth beyond words, redefining or limiting the end to justify the means. They only serve to strengthen

---

[214] *Tantric Jnana* is the yoga of nonduality in consciousness and energy.

the impression that the chosen method is the right one, the best or the fastest route. It is a misplaced kind of motivation:

- The blinder kinds of *Bhakti Yoga* may lead to unhealthy identification with a particular form chosen to represent the essentially formless divine cosmic Self. Love can make us blind and that may also happen in spiritual devotion. 'My God is better than your God' then becomes the issue and produces all well-known group-ego related distortions of the absolute truth in religion. This problem is rather inherent to monotheistic religions, but of course also in polytheistic Hinduism, devotees of a particular form of the divine may show a tendency to place that form above all others. The same is true for those that choose a more human object of worship, such as in Buddhism or in Guruism. Nevertheless in polytheism, respect for all forms of the divine is rather inherent[215].

- *Karma Yoga* may also defy its very objective, when the result of our selfless service is wrongly attached to as a reality. The *Karma* Yogi should not forget that we do this service in order to solve some of the problems caused by our own ego. That service may consist of addressing some of the more practical problems of others, but these are not the real problems. The only relatively real problem is the ego which we all have, and all other problems are an illusion. Thus our selfless service is not a reality, and neither is the result of it. The best *Karma Yoga* lies in sharing spiritual teaching, as it helps others more significantly in reducing their ego problem. Second best is to help those who are really so imbalanced, that applying spiritual understanding and moving

---

[215] I once did a survey of over 100 Hindus, asking for their favorite deity and its relation to others. Not one person could be found that did not confirm all Hindu deities being in essence the same.

forward on the path seems to become nearly impossible.

- *Jnana Yoga* has the tendency to become very intellectual and all too solar, suppressing feelings, as explained before. It largely rests upon mere conviction and will power, keeping our head above the waters of illusion twenty four hours a day. This is in truth such a tough stance, that any other idea may be seen as being in competition with it. Hence disdain for any other path or practice easily develops, which may not only confuse and alienate others. It can also keep us from following some other paths that might be very useful to pursue. Especially as people encounter the more subconscious blockages, it can lead to stagnation and even a kind of cynicism or depression.

- *Ashtanga Yoga* has meanwhile taken many different forms in so many schools all over the world. Preference for only one or a few of the eight limbs has led to some very limited interpretations. Especially in the West, emphasis on health and outer beauty brought a performance of *Yoga* postures that stimulates the ego rather than reducing it. Another issue is that the first limb of avoiding that which removes peace tends to become a kind of generalized morality, even though it must always be a personalized practice, such as in the case of sexual abstention. Attachment to the bliss gained in meditation may lead to an extreme sensitivity for any outer disturbance of the peace, while the true disturbance lies inside. Identification with the yogic powers that may come through the practice of deep meditation is probably the most powerful trap, leading to an extremely inflated ego.

- In *Tantra Yoga* one's understanding may be clouded in too much mystery, getting confused by the many details that are typical in tantric practice, and losing natural intuition as a result. As with other paths, it may produce disrespect towards other cultures and traditions. As in *Ashtanga*, whatever powers are acquired may likewise be confused with the real objective of yoga, which has nothing to do with having more or less power. Purely tantric powers are not one's own anyhow, as they rest upon relationships with beings in the spiritual world. And even the true yogic powers gained through *Ashtanga* or *Kundalini Yoga* rely directly upon the Self, so the ego cannot claim them either. Some *Tantric*s of course have given *Tantra Yoga* a bad name by misusing the truly sacred knowledge of *Tantra* for selfish reasons. *Tantra* can be used for a more worldly purpose or for a more spiritual, yogic purpose, yet some use it for harming others, stealing from them, manipulating them. One must be always aware that not every *Tantric* is a yogi, and that to have some special powers does not make a person a saint. Moreover, many people 'behave' in part out of fear of retribution. If particular powers allow us to escape any retribution, our moral backbone is truly put to the test.

For every yogi, there is a unique yoga. While the destination is the same for all, the path depends on where we are coming from in terms of our individual types, talents and blockages. However useful it surely may be to become deeply connected to a particular yoga tradition, we should always remain open minded. One practice hardly ever opposes another – the true relationship between different practices is by nature complementary. To overly cling to one tradition against all reason and need, is another ego game. May the fundamental understanding that all paths and practices originate from the seeds within the Self, bring a deeper sense of connection between the followers of different traditions.

11
KEEP IT SIMPLE

Exploring *Tantric Advaita*, we have expanded our understanding of the rather simple nonduality of the unmanifested Self, with the relative complexity of the nondual energies that exist within manifestation. Likewise, the simple technique of 'just being' has been complemented with a rather dazzling variety of other practices, which the yogic traditions created in support of it. They balance different energies of our manifested being, in order to produce the nondual energy of the Self. That may truly be seen as an invitation or the perfect excuse for too much side-tracking into all kinds of complex activities, causing one to forget the true goal, the actual practice, which is quite simple indeed.

The first way to avoid that mistake is to always end whatever practice with the non-practice of pure being. That should definitely always be the cherry on the cake of any meditative sequence. In as far as the preceding practices are suitable, they will facilitate that experience of pure beingness most easily. It is how we can truly collect on the efforts made.

The second way is to always first counter any unpleasant feeling with whatever bliss of the Self we can generate, withdrawing into the silent, formless, blissful observer of the now. If that works, fine. If it doesn't, all other techniques come into play to generate more nondual energy, depending on whatever imbalance is experienced.

Simply put, every practice should start and end with the Self. While working with our energy often produces very direct results, some people are entirely too focused on it. They may be seen to frantically search for some reason for their unhappiness in the food they ate, the energy of some place or the disturbed emotions of another, while forgetting that simple withdrawal may often be enough to deal with all of that. When an unpleasant feeling is gone, there is not much use in knowing why it was there in the first place. Only when it persists, we are free to seek its cause and take it out by the root.

It is advised by most traditions to keep it simple by mastering at least one technique that works on the energy level. Whether it involves breath, a *mantra*, or the cleansing of our energy channels, it does not matter. Whatever technique we have found that really works for us, we exercise it until we become as good at it as let's say Roger Federer is at tennis. It is truly not possible for a book to tell us which practice will best suit us. I hope this one gives enough insight to try out some things, and only then our ideal practice may be revealed. The complexity of individual existence is truly beyond intellectual comprehension, while it is definitely not beyond direct experience.

Experience leads to conviction and from there to real practice and mastery. Then we will really have an energetic tool at hand, which can bring us back to the nondual energy of the Self anytime we feel the need. Other energetic techniques may still be useful from time to time for dealing with some particular cause or a recurring karmic imbalance. This one master technique should in any case be able to temporarily bring back balance, even if it may not always address the cause of such imbalance. This mastery is obtained by intensively exercising it outside of life and then also really using it in life.

This chapter on 'Keeping it simple' is obviously short. Using any techniques beyond non-doing and that key master-technique on the energy level comes down to three subjects, which correspond to the remaining chapters: good habits, meditation and life.

12

GOOD HABITS

Habits are great to keep our energy more balanced the simple way. While it may take some study and effort to create them, once we have developed them, they require little attention. Habits are not very fashionable, with people loving the feeling of being free to do whatever they want, whenever, wherever. We are free to bear the consequences as well. We can let the energies of life play with us, or we can play with them. Just as in raising kids, good habits provide healthy structures to our lives. They allow us to keep various aspects of ourselves in control, rather than being controlled by them. That is the real freedom.

Instead of having to repeatedly think about when we want to do something, we only have to think about it once, if we can make a good habit out of it. So if we feel that some daily chanting of *Bhajans* would do us so much good, why not accommodate for it in our daily schedule? The alternative is to have to go through some decision-making process about it every single day, which probably means we will often skip it, depending on mood and circumstances at that moment. Usually, we have to take the needs and schedules of others into account, which is again easier to manage with some regularity. Habits are particularly important in maintaining some regular healing or cleansing therapies, as without such regularity many of these Self-help home remedies that keep the doctor away, may not properly work[216].

One of the most important good habits is of course to daily cook food that maximally supports our worldly and spiritual objectives. That means food which is fresh and natural, gently cooked with herbs and spices, light and nourishing, balancing the six tastes, the three *Dosha*s and the three *Gunas*[217].

Many good habits will bring our energy more in tune with some major natural cycles, while their absence often means we may be doing the right thing at the wrong time. We can ignore the nature of the cosmos, or work along with it. The most relevant cycles are those of sun and moon, which means our habits should be based upon the natural rhythm of day and night[218], as well as on the moon cycle.

DAILY RHYTHM

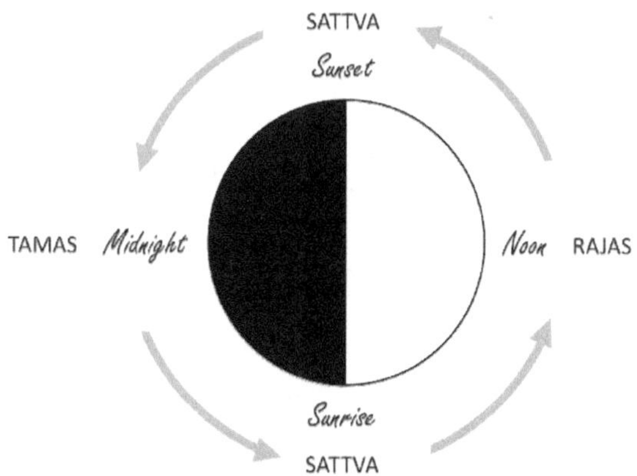

ill. 28. - The Gunas of the Day.

---

[216] In *Ayurveda*, many cures are said to have completed their work only after 40 days of consecutive use.

[217] As discussed in Chapters 7 & 8.

[218] See also 'A Daily Yoga Rhythm' on youtube.com/youyoga.

Sattvic activities belong to the early morning, as that energy quite naturally dominates from about 90 minutes before sunrise to maximally 3 hours after sunrise. During the day, the *Rajasic* energy will be in support of more forceful solar activities, doing our job. Sunset then offers a short interval where again the *Sattvic* energy is more available. After sunset and during the night the *Tamasic* energy dominates.

One of the most spiritually fruitful decisions on daily rhythm is to start the day with peace giving and inspiring *Sattvic* activities. Reserving more me-time in the early morning when the energy is fresh and calm, makes it so much more rewarding. Many have their free time mostly in the evening, when we are usually already quite exhausted and stressed from the *Rajasic* activities of the day. This mostly results in a kind of passive entertainment, which is only somewhat distracting, but will not be very nourishing, relaxing or stimulating.

Many people sleep for as long as possible, jumping out of bed and running off to work shortly after. If we want to have a stressful day, that is exactly how to start it. It is advised to allow our system to wake up slowly and reserve one to three hours every morning for meditation, yoga, artistic expression, cozy togetherness and whatever else brings us more in tune with the energy of the Self. It will then be much easier to keep connected to the Self throughout the day.

While we may not always have the freedom to live like this, getting up early is the key. As most adults tend to sleep quite long and lose a lot of energy in intensive dreaming during the last few hours of lying in bed, having more quality me-time in the early morning is certainly possible. Sleeping less and meditating more usually brings an experience of having more energy rather than less[219].

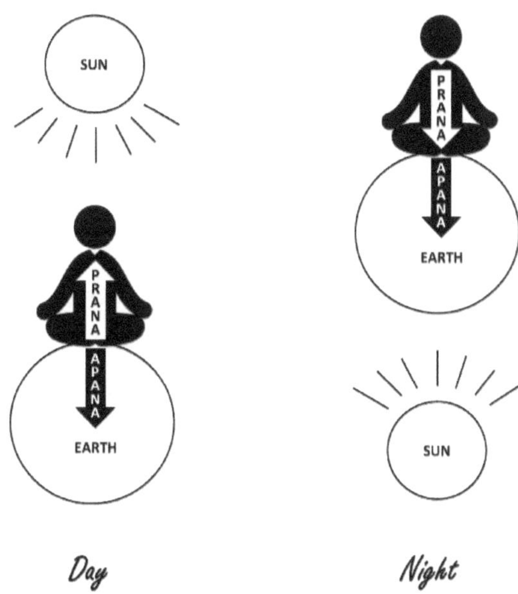

ill. 29. - Impact of Day & Night on Prana & Apana.

Getting up before sunrise offers so many advantages. A major objective here is having regular bowel movements soon after waking, so that *Apana* and all waste materials can leave the body before the natural thinning of the blood starts[220]. *Apana* is pulled downwards by the gravity of the Earth, while *Prana* is attracted by the gravity of the Sun. Then with the rising of the sun above the horizon[221], our vertical position assures that the *Prana* and *Apana* will be separated without

---

[219] Adults do not all need to sleep 8 hours a day. For many, 6 to 7 hours is sufficient and as we get older or meditate more, that may be even less.

[220] This happens at about 10 to 20 minutes before sunrise and brings a strong recirculation of both nutrients and waste materials.

[221] This auspicious time is called '*Brahma Mahoorta*' or the time of Brahma, as well as '*Amrit Bela*', the time of the nectar of life.

an excess of *Apana* polluting the *Prana*. As a result, not only our physical body, but also our vital energy will be purer during the day.

To already be meditating at the moment of sunrise is particularly auspicious, as we may then benefit from the natural balance the sunrise brings to the solar and lunar energies, generating the neutral energy by balancing nostril dominance[222]. The further we live from the equator however, the more sunrise times in summer and winter will vary, which should then not become too much of an obsession[223].

Ideally, we should move from sleep into meditation as soon as possible, except when we really have lots of time in the morning. Then we first might do some more physical stretching, to prepare the body for the lack of movement when sitting in meditation. Before meditation, it is advisable to avoid any unnecessary excitement, including coffee, media and conversation. A short morning walk, looking at flowers, sitting by a natural fire, cleaning throat and nostrils[224] and gently washing face, mouth, hands and feet[225] are considered beneficial[226].

Following meditation, more intensive physical exercises are logically followed by bathing and changing clothes. Only then our energy is really ready to formulate some intentions for the coming day, plan ahead and maybe perform some devotional ritual in support of it. Some great but light breakfast enjoyed in togetherness logically comes next. Whatever free time remains can be spent in artistic

---

[222] As seen in Chapter 7.

[223] In Belgium where I live, sunrise times vary from 4:45 to 8:45 am, so to center the morning schedule around sunrise is simply not workable for part of the year.

[224] The practice known as '*Neti*'.

[225] This is called the '*Panch Shnanam*' or the 'five baths', washing face including mouth, two hands and two feet.

[226] See for many more details on 'The Glory of Waking Up': 'Dhanwantari' by Harish Johari, Rupa Publications India 2001..

expression, making music, studying scriptures, journaling, etc. Then comes in fact the most obvious moment if desired to check out what is happening in the world through the media of our choice, before actually moving more into the world and work[227]. The above is just giving some idea of what morning schedule might work, while each has to make up their own mind about it, and it may vary from day to day.

However, everyone has experienced how much easier it is to wake up refreshed if one always wakes up at the same time. That is the case for many other aspects of our daily rhythm, improving sleep, digestion, bowel movement and meditation. Falling asleep will be so much easier if we always retire at the same time. Another timing that determines so many other things is that of daily meals.

The effect of digestion on our energy is quite strong and proper digestion cannot happen if eating is followed by too much movement. Any serious physical exercise should always happen before meals, that is before breakfast, lunch or supper[228]. Digestion may be supported by gentle walking afterwards, aiding the work of gravity. The time after meals is ideal for more relaxed physical or mental activity, togetherness and some entertainment. Any inspired mental activity is easier when we are not under the *Tamasic* influence of digestion.

Sleeping shortly after meals is a recipe for constipation and gastritis. In-between snacks are best to be avoided, so our digestive system has the time to clean itself in between meals. That strongly reduces the presence of waste materials in our system that may

---

[227] Though under much pressure from the more Western views on work, traditionally in India people went off to work at around 10 am, even though getting up quite early.

[228] In too many yoga centers, the lack of communication on this subject is a grave error.

pollute our mood[229], as well as create health issues such as atherosclerosis. In case of physical, mental or emotional imbalance, detoxification may be essential to recover balance. Both yoga and *Ayurveda* offer many means to that end[230].

While breakfast should be light in support of the sattvic morning activities, it may need to contain enough energy to support the activities during the day. Any heavier meals can be most easily digested if eaten before sunset. Heavy meals taken after sunset may stimulate the more *Tamasic Rasas* such as fear or depression. Generally speaking, after sunset is the ideal time for some light entertainment in order to avoid unpleasant emotions.

Before going to sleep, at least one hour should be reserved to properly calm down our system, considering also how too much light before sleep may disturb the sleeping process[231]. Foot massage and combing the hair before retiring can help to induce sleep. If sleep is chronically disturbed, it represents a major wakeup call that stress needs to be somehow reduced or some more profound healing is required. For those that can afford it, meditation is equally possible towards the middle of the night, when the world outside has become really quiet, including the common mind-field.

THE MOON CYCLE

Perhaps the most overlooked natural cycle in modern society is that of the moon, even though its effects are visible everywhere in nature. At full moon the earth is moving more or less between the sun

---

[229] Called '*Amma*' in Sanskrit.

[230] Among which are the famous '*Panchkarmas*', various fasts and also many yoga postures and breathing exercises.

[231] The impact of all kinds of lights and screens on Melatonin is well known also the West.

and the moon. During this time, the gravitational pull of sun and moon happen in opposite directions. As a result, the solar and lunar energies are less in balance. One might say that around full moon the gap between the lunar and solar hemispheres of the brain, between feeling and thinking, becomes wider. This imbalance means that the emotional energy becomes more pronounced, increasing the possibility for outbursts of anger and anxiety, but also allowing for great sex and partying.

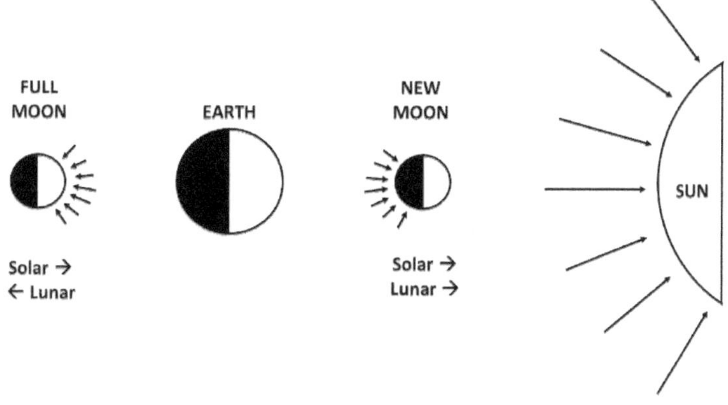

ill. 30. - Impact of the Moon Cycle on Solar & Lunar Energy.

At new moon, the sun and the moon are more or less on the same side of the earth. Then sun and moon pull in the same direction and solar and lunar energies are more balanced. The emotional energy becomes less pronounced, which may create more calmness, but might increase feelings of sadness, worrying and depression, because of lack of passion and confidence.

Respecting the moon cycle in our planning will greatly enhance the fruits of our endeavors[232]. For example, never try throwing a great party on new moon, because people's energy will be low. If some

---

[232] The moon cycle has been in my agenda for over 30 years.

family dinner however poses the danger of too much quarreling, a new moon timing might be ideal to help avoid that.

It is advisable to take the moon cycle into account in varying our meditation sequence. Around the new moon we can more easily achieve deep peace in meditation, while our daily discipline and the phase of concentration might be weakened by lack of will power. That phase should then maybe take more time, step by sure step increasing our concentration. Around the full moon, meditation is more likely to be needed to reduce stress and might at times not achieve much more than that. We may then need to set aside more time for relaxation prior to our meditation, while our will power of concentration will be stronger. All that obviously depends on how accomplished we are in relaxation, concentration and meditation. If we can achieve deep meditation around the full moon, it may bring highly valuable experiences of the spiritual dimensions.

As our will power and passion fluctuate during the moon cycle, it strongly affects our decision making. Especially any decisions on new spiritual disciplines should happen at the right time. The new moon provides the calmness for wise reflection in preparation of any decisions, but our will power is then often too weak to make any really courageous decisions. Any changes made or decisions taken on new moon itself are said to be not lasting, impotent. Important decisions should happen within the period starting a few days after a new moon, till a few days before the next full moon. As the emotional energy and passion continues to rise towards full moon, any decision that affects for example the daily rhythm will be easy to respect. Thus any new habit will already be well established by the time the full moon rises.

Ideally, making important decisions should be avoided for a few days around the full moon. They may easily turn out to be too emotional, too drastic, overestimating our abilities, blowing our desires out of proportion. Likewise, it is not the right time to engage in important emotional discussions with partners, friends, family and co-workers. During the period between full moon and new moon, all big decisions should be avoided if possible and the ever-decreasing energy should be used to maintain whatever disciplines we decided upon before full moon. It is an ideal time to finish any project or do some maintenance. If possible, the time around new moon should be empty of objectives and too much work.

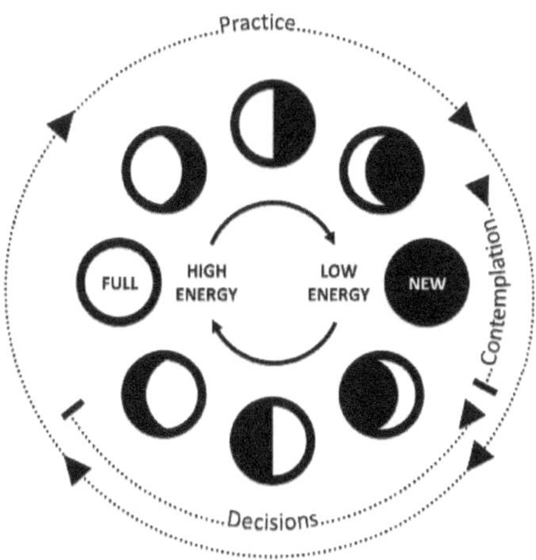

ill. 31. - Synchronizing Decisions with the Moon Cycle.

The new and full moon are special times when the connection to the spiritual world is more pronounced. Ancestor rituals are particularly fruitful on a new moon, as the ancestors will be more calm and receptive. Other rituals directed at higher energies are not very effective during this time, as these are then more turned away from the Earth dimension. The full moon on the other hand is ideal for working with higher spiritual energies. The emotionality is then particularly suited for *Bhakti Yoga* and definitely also for fire rituals[233].

Women have their own moon cycle of menstruation of course, which is said to be ideally synchronized with the actual moon cycle. Lacking any direct experience, I prefer not to comment on the subject, except in saying from indirect experience that a woman's cycle may be extremely important to respect in any planning.

OTHER NATURAL CYCLES

As work usually affects how each week is being lived, some weekly habits are therefore logical. They may be especially needed to assure regularity in some activities that we feel are important for our mental, emotional and spiritual health. Any such practice that is performed less than weekly will have little effect, even if of course an occasional 'special' may be particularly useful and fruitful.

The four seasons of course each have their own particular energy, which is best respected. The need for food and sleep in winter increases, while in summer we may need to drink considerably more. Food fasts are then most logical both during spring and summer. Outdoor activities tend to be replaced with more indoor activities during winter, which greatly increases the need for breathing exercises. Indoor air has less Prana, depending also on proper ventilation. Countering important astrological changes may require particular practices, which in Hindu culture are largely assured through their extensive calendar filled with spiritual festivals and observances.

---

[233] Known as '*Havan*', '*Homa*' or '*Agnihotri*'.

AVOIDABLE HABITS

While we can strengthen good habits by ensuring regularity, we can weaken the less desirable habits by breaking their regularity. As long as we feel that we cannot totally let go of them, we should not allow them to further take root. Breaking the timing of any bad habit is advised, as well as regularly fasting from any such habit for as much time as we can manage. This is about a weekly food fast or one day a week without sugar, avoiding always smoking at particular times, not having alcohol every evening, not giving in to the need for that huge cake every Sunday, and so on.

Unhealthy habits are usually supported by unhappiness. It is generally advised to first promote healthier habits that will increase our happiness, before tackling any of the avoidable habits.

13
MEDITATION

When meditation is taught, usually only one method is put forward, which really makes no sense at all. Everyone is different. Some people are rather emotional and need a different approach than people who are very rational. Some people are hyperactive and need more time to relax. Some people concentrate very easily, but have difficulty to let go of control, which is required in the later stages of meditation. And other people have a tough time concentrating, but once they achieve concentration, it is very easy to surrender and enter a more peaceful kind of meditation with less willpower involved. Some people are more visual while others prefer to work with words, with *mantra*, with the auditory part of our brain. Some simply adore *mantras* and other exotic things from India. Some prefer something more abstract like the Self, the pure beingness, breath or something more personal or belonging to their own culture.

So, all these differences and preferences need to be considered. But we can try not to be too opinionated about different meditation practices, not have our ego stand in the way. Whatever might work, we can just give it a try, without having any prior fixed ideas. Once we try something, then we will know if it works for us, which is then a matter of fact, not of opinion.

WHY MEDITATE?

There is a short-term and a long-term goal to meditation. The most direct goal is simply to bring more peace in our lives. We all want peace, but we seldom give peace a chance. It is not in the nature of peace to ask for attention. People, jobs, feelings, belongings, etc. are all asking for our attention, but peace is not. So, only if we give it some attention, some place in our daily rhythm, we can find it. Meditation brings the power of peace into our relationships, work and health. It enhances the quality and clarity of life. We become more of a master of ourselves. We become a master of our mind and its emotional energy. That way we can grow, generating more and more connection to the nondual energy of the Self. From the very first day of starting some meditation practice, peace will increase, as long as we do not allow frustration to enter the game.

The long-term goal of meditation is to bring us truly inside, where we ourselves reside as pure conscious energy, always in peace and bliss. True deep meditation will enable us afterwards to connect to that inner Self whenever in life we want to, but that first requires at least one or a few very deep experiences of it. Once we have had that entirely pure experience of the Self, it will become quite easy to remain peaceful whatever happens. Deep meditation in the long run thus truly realizes the principal objective of yoga: to be happy whenever we want, independent of what happens.

This is a long-term objective, because to get some actual deep meditation experience[234], where body consciousness really disappears, takes a lot of work and time in most people. It is a process in which we grow in our practice, and then slowly, slowly the real

---

[234] '*Samadhi*' or Absorption.

absorption into the Self starts happening, which brings a huge transformation of our personality. Deep meditation may remove many subconscious blockages, frustrations and things that are stopping us from being whom we want to be and who we truly are. Meditation is not the goal of yoga, but certainly the path of yoga passes through meditation. Passing off this process as just a little dwelling in silence, while still remaining fully aware of our environment and our thoughts, is not doing the real objective of meditation much credit. That phase actually belongs to the start of the fifth limb of *Ashtanga Yoga*, when we become ready to withdraw inside.

LEARNING HOW TO MEDITATE

For many, meditation is a major obstacle and that is really a pity. Everyone can learn how to meditate. We only need to regularly devote some time to it, properly know what we are trying to achieve, and adapt our techniques following our experiences. I have been meditating for more than 40 years and I am still learning. There is always some kind of evolution. There are at all times things to learn and to try out and, in this way, the practice just evolves. It gets a lot easier quickly for most people, but still there are layers upon layers of learning. This is especially true once we start reaching deep meditation, which has so many stages. These are layers within ourselves, as they exist within the many dimensions of the cosmos, which we have to encounter, dissolve and let go.

First of all, this learning requires doing. Too many people are thinking about meditation instead of doing it, so I must emphasize some daily meditation habit. Only by regular exercise we can move forward. Whatever is written here are just words on paper until someone gives it a try. Once we have truly practiced some technique and can talk about it in our own words, only then we have truly gained the skill and the understanding, and thinking about it makes sense.

Daily practice is equally important to remain at peace with ourselves. If we practice, we can more easily accept that we are imperfect. As long as there is no practice, spirituality is all just stories going on in our mind. Then very easily we become dissatisfied with ourselves and even turn away from the spiritual path, because it just creates too many problems in the 'spiritual ego'[235]. But if we practice regularly, then we know that slowly, slowly we are moving forward. A work in progress does require work. Some of us are very busy during the day and have only a short time for daily practice, but even then we can be patient, as long as we make the best use of the time available. Somehow, if we make the effort, then life provides the time and then some, to do even more.

Learning how to meditate involves making choices. It is important to point out that, while everybody is so different and unique, the actual process is somewhat the same for everyone. Only when we have insight in the general process, we can make our own choices within this process. What needs to happen is basically the same for all while, how we can do it is totally individual.

Starting with a clear intention, we relax whichever part of us that feels tense in body, breath and the senses. Then we willfully withdraw inside and concentrate our attention on the meditation object, until we reach the stability of effortless meditation. We then remain in that state, until naturally the doer disappears, and deep meditation happens. This chapter tries to sketch the process and point out the

---

[235] We can get too attached to our spiritual achievements, and even though these are beneficial attachments, it may create many problems.

main choices. To dig into the subject, a separate book is needed[236].

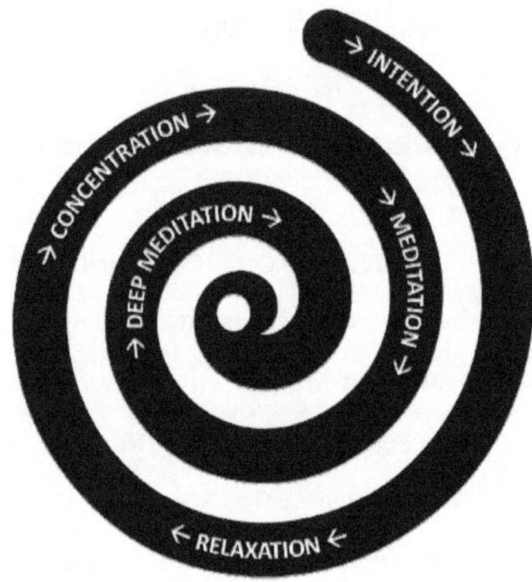

ill. 32. - The Process of Meditation.

MEDITATION INTENTION

Meditation means to let go of everything else. All day, we are so involved with everything and everyone and then suddenly we sit on our meditation mat and just expect to let all of that go. That is why it is beneficial to formulate a clear intention, affirming to ourselves that we want to meditate and why we want to do it.

Expressing a proper intention actually means to contemplate a little. In contemplation we not only think, "Now I want to meditate", but rather we try to feel it, experience the value of it. By trying to sense our intention from a deeper level, it gains power. It is advised to phrase our intention inside and then let it hang in our inner space, focus on it without thinking about it. This way, the power of its feeling will come

---

[236] Until then, you can watch the series of 12 'Personalized Meditation' classes on youtube.com/youyoga, of which a book version is in progress.

forward, and we can move into the practice with full conviction.

Formulating some intention is also about having a meditation plan. This avoids spending too much time thinking about what we are going to do, while we are meditating. Our particular meditation sequence of that day must be clear, including the time given to each part. That means we can be flexible along the way, but we should not jump around from one practice to another like a rabbit. It is definitely advisable to set a time for our practice, otherwise mind will easily find some excuse to stop prematurely. When reciting *mantras,* the use of a rosary[237] is traditional, but one might also use some gentle alarm signal. Keeping a particular sequence steady for some period of time[238], engages the rather miraculous power of repetition.

Our intention may be supported from the spiritual world, by investing in a small ritual at the beginning of each meditation. Asking help for a more fruitful meditation from whatever divine energies we feel attracted to, definitely works. It is another obvious way through which we can have some experience of the spiritual world. That help mostly comes as relaxation, and when we reach the stage of deep meditation, when we ourselves withdraw to the spiritual world. Concentration is our will, our freedom, our intention, so we can never ask for that. This kind of ritual might take just a minute or two, minimally offering some light, some water, some leaf or flower, some incense and some *mantra* or prayer, following the same tantric science explained for ancestor rituals[239].

The following examples may be inspiring to formulate a more personal meditation intention. It is advisable to keep it short, no more

---

[237] *'Mala'* in Sanskrit, which means 'garland'.

[238] Different periods are indicated: 11, 27, 40, 54 up to 108 days or more.

[239] See Chapter 10.

than a few lines that we learn by heart and probably silently repeat at the beginning of each meditation session:

In this moment, I accept the world as it is.
In this moment, I accept myself as I am.
In this moment, only peace matters.

I take this moment to transform myself.
In essence, I am not different from anybody else.
Transformation only takes time and effort.
I am a great work in progress.

Every day I take a step forward.
Every day, I allow peace to work its magic.
In this moment, I will let peace be.
In this moment I return to my divine essence.

I accept that my body and mind resist holding still.
With patience and loving kindness,
I will bring them to silence.

Let the enlightened energies in the universe help me.
Let my divine essence come forward.
Let there be peace, peace, and only peace.

RELAXATION

Depending on how relaxed we feel or not, often also related to how stressful our day or night has been, we may need some relaxation of our whole being before starting to meditate. Whichever part of our being that is not relaxed will annoy us in the next phases. If the body is not relaxed, it is going to hurt and will take us out of our concentration. The same goes if our emotional *pranic* energy is not in balance or when our senses seem overly sensitive[240].

First posture and breath need to be stable, so that we become like a softly breathing, effortless statue. If we cannot sit comfortably, painlessly, how can we meditate? Developing a stable and comfortable sitting posture is too wide of a subject to be fully addressed here. For sure, meditating on a chair or while lying down cannot take us into deep meditation. As then we will lose body consciousness, we will either drop off the chair or fall asleep where we lie[241]. Yet, everyone can find a way to sit comfortably by using props in the right places, assuring that our spine is relatively straight. This way the energy can easily move upwards, and we can truly sit comfortably on our spine and sitting bones.

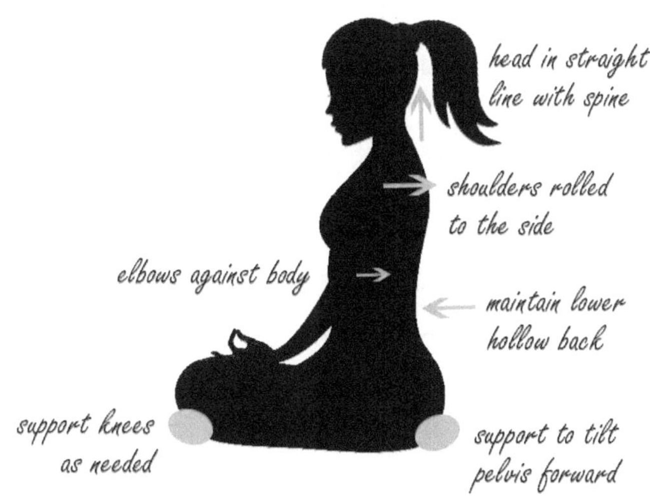

ill. 33. - Sitting on the spine in meditation.

---

[240] Body, *Prana* and Senses correspond to limbs 3, 4 and 5 of the eight limbs of *Ashtanga Yoga*.

[241] Some very advanced yogis have been known to go into deep meditation (*Samadhi*) while lying down, which is often done when the Samadhi is meant to stay for days or weeks. So, it is possible and also the ultimate objective of the practice of 'yogic sleep', known as '*Yoga Nidra*'.

Most people need to sit on the side of some cushion or rolled-up blanket, so that the pelvis is tilted forward. This way, we maintain a slightly hollow lower back, so that our spine seen from the side shows the flexible S-curve. It will allow us to comfortably sit on our spine, like on a spring. As long as the knees do not touch the floor, we use some cushion to support them, so our leg muscles can relax, and the knees gradually come down[242]. The head should be slightly tilted forward and gently drawn upward, like as if on a string. The shoulders should not hang towards the front, rather they are rolled to the side planes. We keep the elbows close to the body, letting our forearms rest on the legs. Once deeper meditation starts happening, our head and body may start leaning into our sitting pose, which is fine.

Holding the body still as a statue helps to silence the mind. Any resulting stiffness easily goes when we start moving again afterwards, which is also true for numb legs. To assure grounding, meditation should happen on a natural material. We can use the movement caused in the body by deeper breathing to fine-tune our posture, sinking further into the most stable pose with every exhale.

While learning different breathing techniques requires a step-by-step approach, after a while the most important aspects of meditative breathing can easily be combined in a single exercise. Breathe slowly and deeply, using breath retention after each inhale, while also applying alternate nostril breathing and *pranic* visualization. A *mantra* can even be added as a counting device to make the breathing pattern more regular. The result of such integrated effort will be a state of calm one-pointedness, and then we can really turn inward.

The whole idea of meditation is to go inside. Things like 'walking meditation' exist as preliminary practices, but if we are truly centered

---

[242] Bringing the knees to the floor may take weeks or months of practice and must not be forced.

inside how can any normal person walk without walking into a wall? Guided meditation may bring us to the inside, yet that is as far as guided meditation can go. As long as we are still listening to someone talking, we are not fully absorbed inside. Some people excel at relaxing everybody by speaking to them, by making them go through certain experiences, leading them into certain visualizations. This is all very good, but if we want to move further, we're on our own.

The relaxation phase can be long or short and finally leads to what people these days call mindfulness. That means the mind is still full of impressions and changes, but we are observing them rather than interacting with them. We are still aware of sounds or thoughts, yet we are somewhat distanced from them, disidentified, which means we are ready to truly concentrate inside.

The senses may also need some purification first, using singing bowls or whatever. The real practice is that while we cannot entirely stop our ears from hearing, we can stop listening. Thoughts then become like fleeting clouds, nothing important. If possible, we hold on to inner silence and let that work for us for a while, before moving onto the next phase of concentration.

CONCENTRATION

Meditation means to stop thinking, but since this is very hard to keep up for most people, at least we can think only one thing and repeat it. To concentrate means to focus on a single object. To visualize the many energies moving through the chakras for example, is still part of the relaxation phase. Choosing our meditation object is quite important, since we are looking to marry a meditation partner that might stay with us for a long time. If we do not feel a particular attraction somewhere, we just try out things until we do. Throughout life our favorite meditation object may change, but some loyalty definitely pays off. The more loyal we are, the more this object becomes part of us, as we become part of it, merging our energies.

Maybe that object will be a *mantra*, or the pure being, a lotus flower, etc. or maybe the combination of a *mantra* and a visual like a *yantra*. As the objective of meditation is the formless Self, many tend towards meditation on a formless object. Yet, it is generally seen as an easier route to concentrate of something with form first, leading towards the formless later[243]. It is mind that needs to be concentrated and mind is all about forms.

Feeling love for our object is obviously very helpful to concentrate on it. It may seem important that it fits into our personal spiritual philosophy. It is especially advisable that the object has some energetic power, so that it not only serves as any object, but will directly help to relax our energy and mind. Here the particular powers of Sound, Space and Time attain their master role, as discussed in the previous chapters. *Mantra*, *Yantra* and *Prana* are the main energetic meditation objects brought forward by thousands of years of yogic experience, among many others.

When we have chosen our meditation object, we need to give it a place within our body. If that does not happen, then mind will tend to move our attention through various parts of the body, reporting on a little pain here, some heat there, etc. Some practitioners are literally chasing mirages within the body, not understanding that any sensation will be naturally stimulated by our attention. Such body scanning may be useful in self-healing, but it is not meditation. Some locations in the body are particularly suited to house the inner space in which we will place the object of our concentration, whether it is

---

[243] Moving from an object with form or '*Saguna*' to an object without form or '*Nirguna*'.

visual or auditory. What will work best largely depends on our personal nature.

More intellectual people, who are primarily into thinking, are advised to choose the third eye. Moreover, the third eye is a great aid in concentration, as our focus on this energy center of the 6th *Chakra* balances solar and lunar thinking. More emotional people, that prefer to feel their way through life, will usually benefit from bringing their object into the heart

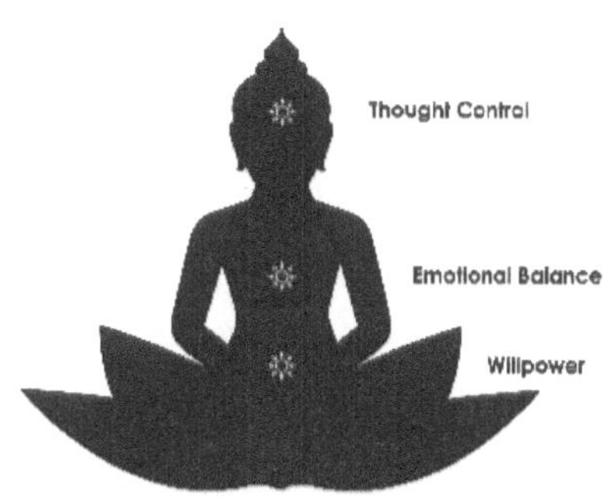

ill. 34. - Centers of Concentration in the Body.

Chakra center, which brings emotional balance. Real doers, that always want to see some action, can best meditate from the navel center, increasing the will power of the 3rd *Chakra*. This is not an exact science, so in case of doubt, just try it out. For example, a 'thinker' might very well benefit from connecting to the heart Chakra.

While the relaxation phase is very nice and entertaining, the phase of concentration is like a mental workout. The effort might even cause our breathing rate to again increase, which is counterproductive to meditation, when it should be avoided. Willpower will be required not to let any other thoughts interfere with our concentration on the object of our meditation. That is where we really teach our mind that we are the boss.

Mind is like a dog. Every dog in some phase of its life needs to be put on a leash and needs to learn to stay close, do whatever the boss is saying. It is the same with our mind. Sometimes, mind needs to be put on a leash, focused and concentrated where we want. It is our tool. Suppose our hands or feet start moving anywhere they want, what are we going to do? Mind easily gets out of control, like some dogs that are not properly trained, creating trouble everywhere if left unattended. So, when we train our mind, it becomes our servant, as it really should be. After a while, it gets so used to it, that it becomes like a very faithful dog. That is also much more agreeable for the dog in the long run.

For sure there are times when mind does not need to be put on a leash, like when enjoying some chocolate, fun conversation or a nice novel. Then we can let mind do what it likes doing, which is to roam around commenting on this and that. That is what mind is for. But the moment we say, 'Stop, come here, focus', it will be used to doing that. To master mind is the first main requirement in becoming a yogi[244], and for that some ego is needed, willpower is needed, doership is needed, perseverance is needed. It is the third step on the stairway to heaven[245], which cannot be skipped.

This is for many a stumbling block because it is hard. Let us just accept from the start, that this will be hard. It will take some time and effort to come to the point where we can do inner *mantra* recitation for example and very few thoughts come in between. If we don't accept that, we will only get frustrated. This phase is actually the easiest thing to teach, but the most demanding thing to do. There is only one answer to any question, which is to return to the object of our meditation.

Fortunately, in the beginning we can ease into it by making the object of our meditation somewhat more complicated, something we can hang on to, a true anchor. For example, we can synchronize silent *mantra* recitation with breath or visualization, giving mind more to do,

---

[244] The Hindu Lord Shiva, master yogi by excellence, is often shown seated on a tiger skin, which represents mind.

[245] See Chapter 8 – Natural Growth.

which will make it easier to stay focused. That is definitely advisable if we experience thoughts disturbing our mind throughout a session, because then the practice really becomes a waste of time. If stopping the avalanche of thoughts requires us to stand on our head or visualize every character of a *mantra*, so be it. Avoid however to focus so hard that the facial muscles become cramped, or you might get a headache. Once the thoughts subside, we again make the object of our meditation as simple as possible. Only that will allow us to move in deeper.

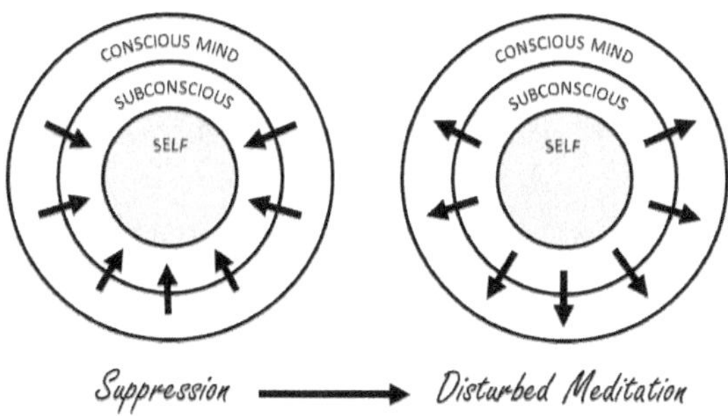

ill. 35. - Suppressed Thoughts Disturbing Meditation.

Some people have a really tough time not thinking, because they have too much to think about. Maybe they have too many projects going on in their lives and need to simplify things first. Or maybe it is because they have been pushing some thoughts away too much. Once we start integrating meditation in our lives, suppressing thoughts and feelings is a luxury we no longer have. Because those are exactly the thoughts that will come to bother us once our meditation starts to work. Then they will be brought into the light while we are meditating. Meditation will then show that this or that subject is something we really need to think about. Maybe it is something from the past, maybe it is some kind of desire or something in our relationships, which really needs our attention. If something really important comes up during our meditation, we set it aside for that moment because we want to stop thinking, but do remember that we will need to deal with it afterwards.

If we are having a hard time concentrating, then the good news is that the next phase will be easier. If this concentration phase of the practice is easy, then the bad news is that the next phase is going to be more difficult. It depends largely on our personality and our balance in solar and lunar energies. To hold on with a lot of willpower, actually anyone can do it, as long as the effort is being made. To hold on with less willpower, with minimal doership, is a lot more difficult, and that is where the phase of real meditation starts.

MEDITATION

When concentration becomes stable, then we are ready to meditate, which basically means the same thing. We are still focusing on one object only, but this should now definitely be a very simple object, which exists totally inside of us. In this phase there can be no more concentration on breath for example, because breathing happens outside of our inner space[246]. We only need to keep breath from accelerating.

So, the object should be inside and it should be held with minimum willpower. If we compare the concentration phase to a firm clenching of the object in our fist, now we have to hold it gently between our thumb and index finger. Meditation is the ultimate feat of

---

[246] People who are so into working with breath that it is hard to let it go, might focus on the inner energy experience of *Prana*.

being simultaneously relaxed and focused, the gentle kind of firm concentration.

This soft focus basically means that we are no longer doing it. It is our mind that is meditating, and we are simply observing this doing from the Self. In this phase any distinction between the meditator, the object of the meditation and the practice of meditation gradually disappears, along with any kind of struggle or effort. Do not resist then to become one with the object, which is not essentially different from the Self.

Just like in the end phase of relaxation when we observe the fluctuations in a distracted mind, we now become the silent observer of a focused mind. All that mind then requires to continue the practice is our full, peaceful attention. Then we just need to persevere, keep doing that. What needs to happen afterwards, happens quite by itself.

DEEP MEDITATION

If we can remain softly concentrated on this one object for enough time, then the next phase of deep meditation comes automatically. This is not something we can do, even if through long practice this non-doing can be mastered[247]. Nobody can 'do' deep meditation, because it is a totally different state of being, where we are no longer in control and thus beyond doing. It comes when we are softly but persistently, confidently but attentively focused on one object only, for a sufficient amount of time. Then through the absence of doer-ship and thoughts, the ego, which is just an idea, the one who is meditating, temporarily leaves the scene. Then we automatically

---

[247] Harish Johari was able to enter deep meditation within minutes and after about 10 minutes we could detect no more breath or heartbeat.

move into the subconscious mind and may finally fully merge with the Self.

Deep meditation is a kind of trance. It may feel like falling asleep, while staying awake. We no longer know that we are sitting there meditating. We are then really absorbed inside, having left the dimension of the physical world and indeed afterwards we feel to have been away somewhere. The conscious mind has stopped functioning, and what happens next is entirely subconscious. We often cannot remember much about it afterwards, yet our smile tells it all. We might not even remember our name for a while, but we know who we truly are, with so much more clarity than before. Laughter, peace and love become Self-evident.

It really goes beyond the scope of this book to really explain what happens there. One might compare it to a kind of hibernation, as both our breath and heartbeat may actually stop[248]. This so-called fourth state of consciousness[249] is entirely beyond what can be described in words, as the conscious mind is no longer present. Yet, remarkable changes will manifest, a shy person losing all shyness, a rather grumpy person becoming a joy to engage with, and so on. However much we can understand about the Self means nothing compared to the true experience and magic of it, which comes in deep meditation.

---

[248] No worry, you will not notice it and if the body cannot hold it any longer, it will 'wake you up'.

[249] Next to the waking state, the dream state and deep sleep.

14
LIFE

Vedic science also offers quite a clear answer to the big 'Why?' question. Why do we live? Why would the unmanifested Self produce the illusion of the manifested universe? The Self is definitely desireless, as the ever-blissful formless beingness that cannot change, having no particular qualities that might change. The logical answer is that the tendency of the Self to manifest is therefore not by intentional desire, but by nature. The ocean makes waves not because it wants to make waves. It just naturally happens.

So, life has no particular purpose beyond itself. The Self manifests for no reason, as the Self exists for no reason. Both the Self and manifestation just exist to exist. And the same then obviously goes for all of us. It is up to us to appreciate life or not. That is truly our only purpose, if we feel the need to have one.

Living nonduality means we do not take life too seriously, seeing it for the illusion that it is. Whatever unpleasantness life brings is therefore also not taken for real. While the search for nonduality makes us turn our awareness away from life, true nonduality thus removes any desire to run away from life. It allows us to lightheartedly play the game, which requires duality, enjoying it while remaining aware of its illusionary nature. In the words of Harish Johari, that is the summum bonum of life as a human being.

In any case, the universe did not manifest out of the Self for the sole purpose of again finding the Self. This quite illogical idea is still very popular within spiritual circles[250]. It would be like a person living in a town who takes the car to drive out on the countryside with the sole and unique purpose of returning home. What does make sense is to take the car, leave the town, enjoy the countryside, and then enjoy arriving back home. Enlightenment in returning to the source may be seen as the last and very enjoyable level played in the game of life, yet that cannot be the unique purpose of life. Life exists to be lived. Who can look at a flower and conclude that it has no purpose in being what it is? That it would not be enough as it is? And what drives people to look upon themselves this way?

Manifestation thus exists for what it actually is, the ever-changing infinite diversity of the full play of Sound, Space and Time, naturally manifesting out of the Being-Knowing-Bliss or *Satchitananda* of the Self. Scriptures point to the *Ananda* or bliss of the Self, as the cause of this desire. It is the energy of time and change without which desire is impossible. Energy, power, desire and goddess are used as synonyms in many vedic scriptures[251]. Thus, the blissful energy of the Self is seen as responsible for naturally creating the ever-changing illusion of the universe, while the consciousness of the Self remains untouched by it. Likewise, we are always free to alternate between playing with the manifested divine energy and staying in the peace of unmanifested divine consciousness, or manage to do both simultaneously. So much unhappiness is created by the belief that we cannot have both.

Manifestation is a grand playground and theatre, unreal as any

---

[250] Some people clearly believe that the Self made a mistake and they want to escape this universe asap.

[251] The word '*Shakti*' especially is used with all these different meanings, even if they also have their own translations.

game, yet potentially quite entertaining. In that possibility of some relatively meaningless divine fun then lies its purpose. All that can be said is that we are free to enjoy it or not. As desires mature, we do add meaning and depth to our performances and entertainment, which leads to ever greater enjoyment. Until the story behind a helping hand, a fabulous dish made from scratch or a song heard in the distance acquire their own kind of magic. Until every second becomes an absolute truth of its own.

We all know to some degree the inherent happiness of the Self. That perfect, subtle flavor of ecstasy naturally becomes our primary desire even in manifestation. Yet, we are then so easily deluded into seeking it primarily outside of us. The path of yoga teaches us how to enjoy manifestation, while still remaining connected to the bliss of the Self inside. From that subtle fine feeling, the beauty of the world is ever revealed in its divine form. This way, the duality between manifested and unmanifested can be dissolved, and we can enjoy life without losing our happiness in the process. If nonduality cannot be a way of life, then what else ?

As we are invited by the very Self to play at life, feel invited simultaneously by that same Self to play at yoga. Anything we do in life can be a practice, whenever we involve some discipline. It pays to always have some such game running, tickling our spiritual growth by questioning some attachment. Enjoy the balancing effects of good habits based upon true insight into the nature of nondual energy. Maintain regular meditation to always stay connected to our divine being. With the Self and our one energetic master technique at the ready, and maybe some ginger and water, we will never be fooled into unhappiness for long. With *Tantric Advaita* energizing our 'sixth sense' of nondual feeling, we bring heaven on Earth.

Please remember though, we are here to enjoy life. Artfully fulfilling desires is one way to get rid of them. In this game of life, there is literally nothing to lose, not even time. Be a *Yogi* yes, but feel free to be a *Bhogi*[252] in at least equal measure. Let a song produce goosebumps. Enjoy the bliss of being alive. All manifestations of Sound, Space and Time in the universe are not only there for reconnecting to the source. Life is a divine show set up from that very source, a spectacle of eternal entertainment.

Since the union of yoga is also found in the ultimate spice of togetherness, love without measure and expectation. Dance this dance of life, mirroring in dynamic balance every partner energy we might meet. Play the divine game of life, knowing it is just a game, no more, but also no less. Be an artist of life, occasionally winking to the spectators, including ourselves.

Ram Ram,

Peter.

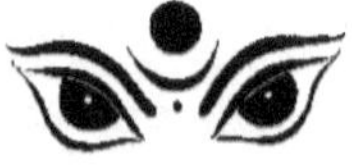

---

[252] As a *Yogi* is a master of Yoga, a *Bhogi* is a master of *Bhoga*, enjoyment.

ADDENDUM

1

The understanding about the nature of nonduality in the Self within the yoga tradition is named *Advaita Vedanta*, where *Advaita* stands for nonduality, and *Vedanta* means a body of knowledge. *Advaita Vedanta* is the most central philosophy of the yogic tradition. *Tantric Advaita* is short for *Tantric Advaita Vedanta*. It represents the ancient body of knowledge (*Vedanta*) on the energetic (*Tantric*) nature of nonduality (*Advaita*).

When we change our breathing to change the energy of our feeling, that is actually *Tantra*, while most people would associate it more with *Yoga*. *Yogic, Vedic* and *Tantric* practices have become so entwined over millennia, that today they are truly inseparable. This way, *Tantric Advaita* or *Tantric Jnana* might also be called *Yogic Advaita* or *Vedic Advaita*, but that would simply bring less emphasis on the subject of nondual energy. This focus precisely makes it so different from more common nonduality teachings.

In India, mysterious practices involving the spiritual world, or the magical use of *Kundalini* energy are seen as particularly tantric. Yoga however can be said to work with both consciousness and energy, while energy is Tantra's more unique domain. In the context of this book, that is how the word Tantra is used. The difference between *Vedic, Tantric* and *Yogic* scriptures seems mostly of interest to historians and scholars. And it is even a lot more complex than that, as there are many other important schools of thought that have contributed to the entirety of spiritual understanding that is very much alive in 'Vedic' culture today[253]. Generally, when discussing some practice or the science behind it, I mostly refer to it in this book as simply *Yogic*. Only when I particularly point out some more energetic or rather occult subject, I refer to it as *Tantric*. Yet generally, if I mention some *Tantric*, *Yogic* or *Vedic* origin of whatever is presented, I never intend to truly distinguish between them.

2

The secrecy and symbolism that are typical for tantric scriptures in part originates with a profound respect towards the rather mysterious divine nature of energy. To claim understanding by making our words very concrete and absolute is seen as disrespectful. I hope not to have made that mistake here, mainly by always pointing out the relativity of whatever can be said. Secrecy was equally needed to protect some of this knowledge from those that might misuse it. Symbolism also caters to the needs of people who through lack of basic education have difficulty comprehending and remembering more abstract explanations. To this day, that is often still the case in more rural or poor areas. Some familiarity with abstract thinking is an advantage of modern education, next to its many disadvantages. Most people can now grasp the meaning of concepts like a void which is full or the basic polarity of energy[254]. It therefore seems an opportune time to translate the ancient tantric mysteries into modern day straightforward language[255].

---

[253] Such as *Samkhya, Nyaya, Vaisheshika, Mimamsa, Vedanta*, etc.

[254] See respectively Chapters 6 and 7.

[255] Nevertheless, their more symbolic or visual expressions may even have superior value.

3

I was truly astonished at the time to discover that Sri Ramana Maharishi was very much involved with the creation of a famous tantric text on the Divine Mother Uma by his student Ganapati Muni. He is even said to have mentally dictated the last 300 verses of it[256]. Equally surprising was his frequent endorsement of an ancient text that very clearly explains *Advaita* philosophy, yet with various forms of the goddess as its central, very tantric representation of the divine Self[257]. Shortly after, I read the last book with the sayings of Sri Nisargatta Maharaj, when just before dying he basically equated the I-Am-ness of the Self to the life force of *Prana*[258]. That really did it, as Nisargadatta is beyond doubt the most unrelenting *Jnana Yoga* teacher I have ever known – though unfortunately not in person.

.I found many more such clues or pointers, like Shankara, the 8th Century father of *Advaita Vedanta,* writing a famous tantric text on the five elements[259]. Also Papaji, student of Ramana and teacher of Mooji and many other modern nonduality teachers, very clearly and quite compassionately referred his students to energetic practices that are complementary to the direct practice of nonduality[260].

As nonduality is the most central yogic philosophy, naturally all traditions and paths have developed their own interpretations. *Tantric Advaita* can then simply be seen as the contribution of the ancient branch of *Tantra Yoga* to the overall understanding of nonduality.

---

[256] 'Uma Sahasram', Sri Ganipathi Muni, Sri Ramanasramam India.

[257] 'Tripura Rahasya: The Mystery beyond the Trinity', Munagala S. Venakataramaiah, Sri Ramanasramam India.

[258] 'Consciousness and the Absolute: The Final Talks of Sri Nisargadatta Maharaj', edited by Jean Dunn, The Acorn Press.

[259] 'Prapanchasara Tantra' by Adi Shankaracharya, Louise M. Finn, Balboa Press.

[260] See for example 'The Truth Is', by Sri H.W.L. Poonja, Red Wheel / Weiser January 1, 2000.

4

Personal experience was essential in bringing me the basic understanding on the nondual seeds of the Self and their primary manifestations in the universe. Yet, many sources for this knowledge exist within a variety of tantric lore, among which the ten *Mahavidyas* or mysteries[261] have been the most revealing to me. They are also ten primordial powers and goddesses. Hence, with the verse found on the one before last page of this book, I offer homage to these ten mysteries that are also essential tantric energies. This is the translation of that verse by Harish Johari:

Kali, Tara, Shodashi, Bhuvaneshwari, Bhairavi, Chinnamasta and Dhumavati, Matangi, Kamala and Bagla Mukhi, are ten great mysteries, which are the secret of all Tantras.

5

It must be clear that nondual words do not exist. When we see the silence, void and timelessness of the Self as nondual, it means that as words they stand unopposed to other words such as sound, space or time. Within the Self, silence, void and timelessness exist by themselves in absolute nonduality to any of their opposite manifestations in the universe.

Our thoughts can thus never truly grasp the reality of nonduality, even though we try. It is also the reason why so many cannot see the nonduality between working with consciousness or working with energy. To our mind it must be one or the other, while in truth both practices are complementary by their very nature.

---

[261] See also 'Tools for Tantra', Harish Johari, Destiny Books 1988 and my 2021 "Mahavidya Mysteries" series on youtube.com/youyoga.

6

The very possibility of nondual energies existing in the manifested universe can be a matter of some intellectual discussion. It seems to depend on the universe being manifested or not.

Also in vedic scripture the universe is said to be in an eternal cycle of birth and rebirth. Each universe is created, maintained and destroyed, followed by a time of non-manifestation[262]. That period of non-manifestation is however a contradiction in terms, as without manifestation there is no time, since there is no change. The time during which the manifested universe would not exist, can thus be seen as the eternity of zero seconds.

The same scriptures also state that during that period of non-manifestation, still there exists a very subtle form of the universe hidden within the most subtle and remote dimensions[263]. Some subtle changes might then still happen within these dimensions, creating time.

As thus the universe can be seen as existing eternally, the primary energies of Aum, Akash and Prana can be regarded as equally permanent.

---

[262] The so-called 'Night of Brahma'.

[263] The most subtle '*Lokas*', see Chapter 9.

ABOUT THE AUTHOR

Peter Marchand teaches Jnana, Karma, Bhakti, Ashtanga and Tantra Yoga. As a personal coach living in Belgium, he guides people from around the world towards happiness, inner peace and deeper meditation. He is a tantric healer, following an ancient Nepalese shamanic tradition. He teaches online and offline, also leading a variety of mantra and bhajan chanting sessions. Until 2020 however, all this was just a hobby, in addition to a busy job.

Originally inspired by his teacher Harish Johari from when he was 20 years old, Peter is one of the founders of Sanatan Society. This association of family and students of Harish Johari was dedicated to spreading his teachings after he left his body in 1999. Peter started teaching in India in 2005. In 2006 he authored "The Yoga of the Nine Emotions", followed by "The Yoga of Truth" in 2007. Around the same time, Peter created his channel on Youtube, where in the following decade he shared over 100 hours of free teaching. Somewhat accidently, Peter wrote the booklet "Love Your Ego" in 2019, stirring his appetite for more. The next year, he left his regular job, now focusing entirely on teaching, writing, healing and coaching.

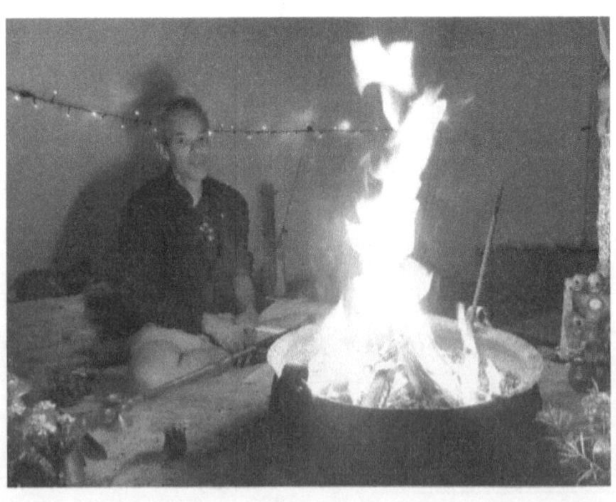

ill. 36. - Fire ritual in the healing Tipi tent of Scheldewindeke - Belgium.

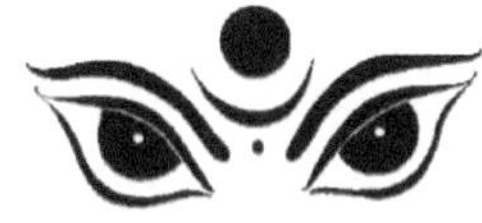

Kali, Tara, Mahavidya Shodashi, Bhuvaneshwari, Bhairvi,
Chinnamasta cha vidya Dhumavati tatha Matangi siddha vidya cha
kathita Baglamukhi eta Dasha Maha Vidya sarva Tantreshu gopitah.

Connect with *Tantric Advaita* through
www.tantricadvaita.org

Enjoy over 100 hours of Peter's free teachings at
www.youtube.com/youyoga

Contact Peter through
www.leela-yoga.org
for personal coaching
and healing through
video calls and visits.

Thank you for posting
your feedback
*on this book at
Amazon & anywhere...
It is truly a great help!*

Peter.

www.ingramcontent.com/pod-product-compliance
Lightning Source LLC
Chambersburg PA
CBHW021143260726

48656CB00024B/1390